Dear Bob,

Thanks for your HDS support and effort.

Bob Kirby

HARD HAT DIVERS

WEAR DRESSES

HARD HAT DIVERS WEAR DRESSES

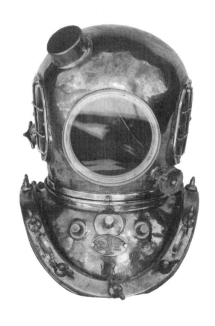

BOB KIRBY

OLIVE PRESS PUBLICATIONS

Front cover painting - Bob Kirby

Typsetting and editing - Lynne Norris

Printed in the United States of America

Olive Press Publications
P.O. Box 99,
Los Olivos CA 93441
805/ 688-2445

CONTENTS

CONTENTS CONTINUED

ACKNOWLEDGEMENTS

As the years rolled along, I became a navy diver, an abalone diver, a boat builder, a fisherman, a seal hunter, a pile driverman, an offshore welder, a construction diver, a machinist, a designer of diving helmets, a mechanical designer, an "actor," and a manufacturer.

This book is based on my life; however, names and incidents have occasionally been altered, not only to make a better story but to keep me out of the courts. They say, "No one can be held accountable for a novel," even if some of it might be true.

The supposedly simple task of writing a book has now consumed five years of my life. Throughout this trauma my wife, Claudia, has supported my purchasing expensive computers that failed, printers that would not print, and me — a husband who had a difficult time dealing with these new-fangled monsters. In order to satisfy my ego, Claudia budgeted, paid the bills, shared the frustrations, and suffered in the process. It is to Claudia that I dedicate this book for, if there is a reward for the effort, it should go to her.

Because I'm dyslexic, I needed help. Many good friends have lent their assistance. George Warner, one of my oldest friends, edited my initial writing efforts and encouraged me to go into greater detail. Mike San Gabriel, a commercial diver, is also a spelling whiz. When the spell checker on my computer did not recognize a buzzword associated with diving, Mike came through. The person who helped me most was probably Jeff Dennis.

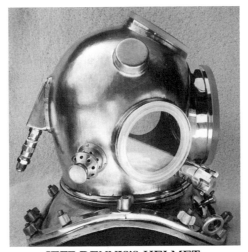

JEFF DENNIS'S HELMET

His skills at rewriting were invaluable and, as payment, I constructed a copper diving helmet for him. Jeff probably got the raw end of the deal.

Ross Saxton and Leslie Leaney also read my manuscript, removing some words and replacing them with others more appropriate. I admit to being at a loss for words, however, and they suggested I eliminate my beloved and frequent swearing. And because I had situations taking place at every turn in history, Ross suggested I tighten up the time lines.

Scrap Lundy, author of *The California Abalone Industry,* encouraged and guided me throughout the process and also lent me many of his photos. Torrance Parker, completing his book *20,000 Jobs Under the Sea,* was another who loaned me photos and inspired me to get my act together. Gene Webb, owner of Orville – my original personal helmet – provided photos of it. Steve Rebuck, by loaning me photos of his dad's boat, the *Laura Belle*, provided accountability for the nutty chapter by that same name.

Leslie Leaney, founder of the Historical Diving Society USA, has earned a special place in my heart. If the chapters he read were particularly awful, he was very quiet; if they were acceptable, he would raise his eyebrows. He was quiet most of the time, and his loan of photos was also invaluable.

Numerous additional friends helped; far too many to list. I can only thank them in a general way, and with all my heart.

INTRODUCTION

The damned crane had continued to settle in the mud. Chances are my entrance under its tracks was now too small to escape through and, adding injury to insult, the old M boat holding my air compressor had slipped its ties and was heading to sea, dragging my umbilical behind. In an effort to align my body through my only escape route, I was forced to unsnap my hose. My mask then flashed out, leaving me trapped with no air. I said a prayer, began to squirm, and eventually ascended to safety.

Among commercial divers, there are few atheists.

Hard Hat Divers Wear Dresses is my autobiography, modified. This is not just my story, however. It is the story of many others − good, bad, indifferent, and/or interesting including Melvin C. Catrel, the dirtiest man in Morro Bay; Bob Long, my boat operator; Laddy Handelman, the founder of Oceaneering; Nasty Ed; "Gentleman" Jerry Todd; and the great sea captain, "Barnacle" Jim Penn. All of these men, and many more, are worthy of a good tale.

Once I found myself in the manufacturing business, I teamed up with Bev Morgan and we created the Kirby Morgan Corporation which later became Diving Systems International and is now Kirby Morgan Dive Systems, Inc., the world's largest manufacturer of commercial diving helmets and masks.

How did all this take place? How could I have traveled from the wrong side of the tracks with almost no education and, in the year 2000, end up the recipient of the John Galletti Award, the highest tribute in commercial diving?

Here, I tell the story of those crazy times, with humor as my medium plus an occasional dose of terror.

Enjoy, Bob Kirby

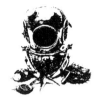

"I'M TODD, BY GOD"

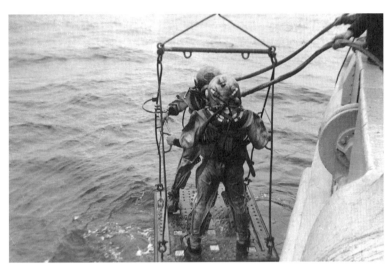

U.S. NAVY QUALIFICATION DIVE

I was in the navy in 1955, working on my assigned ship, the sub-tender *Nereus*, where I was a welder, metal smith, and second-class diver. I had long since earned my third-class rate and was assured there would be no more mess duty. Because I was a diver, and a rather good one I might add, I enjoyed a dip several times a week in San Diego's shipping lane where our large ship was anchored. During an ebb tide, this dip was transformed into a prolonged swim in San Diego's sewer, as this large city's waste ran first into the bay, and then out to sea. It was here that we divers, fifteen in all, labored to accomplish underwater repairs to the flotilla of submarines that were tied against the steel sides of our five-hundred-foot ship.

While aboard this massive, floating workshop, we enjoyed a four-day liberty — three-days-in-four off in the evenings, and three-in-four weekends away, as well. This coming Saturday was one of my weekends aboard, and I would be accompanied by three of my best diving shipmates, Chief Otho "Cress" Cressy, Ed Lawler, and Gene Harless.

Chief Otho Cressy was our master diver. Otho, rather short in stature, had an endless grin. Though he was somewhat awkward on deck, he was a fish in the water and a darned good mechanic as well. Ed Lawler was my direct boss in the shipfitter shop. Ed was a first-class metal smith and a first-class diver. He lacked Cressy's flamboyant personality, but he made up for this with his sincerity and fairness.

The last of our diving rat pack was Gene Harless, a second-class pattern maker.

Because of his strength, excellent abilities, and attitude, Gene had been pried away from his wood shop by Cressy. Gene and I usually worked together as a diving team. (Gene and Cressy have remained my friends over the past forty-five years; Lawler, on the other hand, has escaped from us and into the unknown.)

This weekend was special because one of our subs, the *Remora*, was to receive a change of command. The present skipper was being transferred and a new captain would be taking his place. Where authority figures are concerned, the navies of the world share the same scenario; the navy is the one place on earth where all authority can be transferred from one individual to another in an instant. It is more than a changing of the guard; instead, a total change in authority takes place. It could be compared to the selection of a new Catholic pope.

The year 1955 was the beginning of the end of the USA's long, Korean peace-keeping operation. Many of our young servicemen and women had been wounded or met their maker during the Korean War, and our flotilla of converted, WWII diesel-powered submarines, The West Pack, was no different. Many had returned to their San Diego home port badly damaged; others did not make it home at all. During the Korean War, our entire diving team would labor around the clock in order to send a sub back to active duty.

The mood of our duty diving team was different this particular day. We were not in a hard-hitting or "damn the torpedoes" frame of mind; no working around the clock. Instead, we were experiencing a rather laid-back approach. Our four duty divers, myself included, stood by in anticipation of making a wad of money during the changing of two submarine propellers. Due to negligent seamanship, this was not an uncommon event after a change of sub commands.

Through the whisper-thin San Diego fog appeared the grey lines of a well-maintained sub. Its crew was standing in perfect attention topside as she was guided into her slot alongside our tender. The four of us were lined up against the handrail of our ship fitters shop as we observed the landing, with our arms and elbows drooped over the steel-pipe railing. Cress had guessed correctly. The new captain was showing off by doing his best to place his boat very close to its sister sub while avoiding the use of heaving lines. Each of us was holding an empty, white, navy-issue coffee cup, and we were grinning from ear to ear, in anticipation of an impending crash between two giant brass propellers, one on the approaching boat and the other on the sub that was tied in place. We had witnessed this very foolish maneuver before and knew the inboard propeller of the *Remora* would come in contact with the outboard wheel of the approaching sub, the *Diadon*. As predicted, there was a dull "clank" as the two screws meshed and twisted together.

Cress winked at us. We would now be blessed with two wheel changes instead of one.   Each change would require twenty hours of work and, because we were paid hazardous duty pay – $5 per hour when on the dive station – our dungaree pockets would swell with each wheel change. Not bad pay in 1955.

As a third-class metal smith, my monthly pay plus my hourly diving hazardous duty fee often brought my total nut to a sizable sum – sometimes two, three, or even four times my base pay. My check often surpassed that of many of our oldest chiefs and young officers.

Eyebrows would raise as the paymaster pealed out my reward in front of the ship's company, and I would laugh all the way to the diving locker. Here I displayed my loot to Metal Smith First Class Madox, nicknamed "The Mad Ox." Madox had a habit of selecting a bottle of Scotch over his duties and he seldom made it to the dive station, much less into the water. He seldom felt the thrill of a fat wallet. Goodness, how Madox hated me.

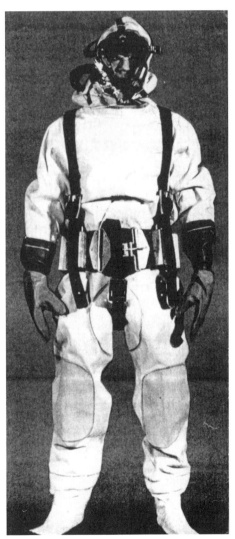

JACK BROWNE BUNNY SUIT

Our diving equipment, "Bunny Suits," supposedly dry dresses, were victims of a long shelf life and were sometimes rotten when they arrived from the manufacturer. When we entered the water, the ensuing leaks could be compared to a cold shower in the ship's head.

The wimpy rubber Jack Browne masks refused to remain in place and lacked electrical communication; instead, we depended upon hose jerks or line signals. Our weight belts were at least thirty pounds, and we had no fins as these necessary devices were not navy-approved for fleet diving, only for the UDT. A slip off our underwater stage meant a twenty-foot trip to the bottom of the bay where we would end in mud — a junk-filled graveyard containing every rusty piece of scrap metal known to man, captured in a field of solidified sewage. (Instead of returning coffee cups to the mess hall, they were scattered below, like oysters in a tide farm. I once ran a long length of six-thread line through the handles and ended up with so many coffee cups, two mess chiefs couldn't have lifted them. My line broke, and the cups remain in the mud today.)

Whenever a dreaded free-fall took place, ear ruptures were not unheard of, and the unpleasant body squeeze, caused by the lack of equalizing air within our flooded suits, formed vivid red lines on our bodies. We looked as if we had been placed before the mast on the good ship *Endeavor*, and beaten with the "cat of nine tails" for smuggling a dozen topless female natives aboard.

Harless and I usually ended up working together, an unorthodox mandate from Cressy which infuriated Chief William Haney, our second master diver who believed second-class divers should only be line tenders. Otho saw things differently and, thank goodness, Harless and I were always called out. This also aggravated the other divers; most of whom were first class and should have had the beginning go at the lucrative underwater work.

My ongoing battle with Chief Haney never ceased. He went by the book, and this included rigging procedures as well as diving. Haney was a poor rigger, and he also had a dim understanding of the underwater task. I did my best to point out his weaknesses and, in retaliation, Haney vowed to rid himself of Third Class Metal Smith Bob Kirby by having me transferred as far away as possible. Because I had done my homework, he was never successful. Many of the ship's complement were in my pocket — before I joined military ranks I had been a journeyman ornamental ironworker. My talents as a civilian afforded me a method for making many good friends, and the list included our executive officer who needed a fancy gate for his home.

At one point in my four-year enlistment, I was determined to attend the first-class diving school in Washington, D.C. In order to achieve this, I was required to spend at least two years of obligated service after dive school graduation. In other words, I would have to re-

4

up for four more years or forget my plan. Then an incident occurred that changed my outlook concerning the military.

I was standing on the afterdeck of the *Diadon*. All her hatches were open and she had been deliberately listed to one side for hull cleaning. This was accomplished by flooding some of ballast tanks on one side only, rolling her hull over, and exposing the green moss on the other side. A team of scrapers would then clean off the unwanted sea life. When this job had been completed, the flooded ballast tanks were blown and the other side was flooded. Cleaning would then resume on the opposite side of the ship.

This particular day, cleaning had been completed on one side, and the order to roll the ship over was announced. However, the first side's ballast tanks were not blown before the opposite side's tanks were flooded and the *Diadon*, losing its buoyancy, started down. As water began pouring into the open rear hatch, I spotted a pair of hands attempting to close it from within the torpedo room. I pried off the sailor's hands and closed the hatch. Before water-tight security was accomplished, I was standing in a foot of water. I began to wade forward in order to secure the sub's other two hatches, one on the foredeck and one in the conning tower.

Agonized screams, whistles and bells pierced the quiet morning, and air was coming from every orifice. Soon the gray shape resumed its position on top of the water. The sub and most of its crew had been saved.

I was approached by the duty deck officer, a new ensign, red-faced and angry as he could be. "Who gave you the order to close the rear hatch?" At first I didn't realize he was serious, but I soon sensed his true intent. Instead of receiving a medal for bravery, I was going to be the recipient of a court martial.

"Sir," I said, "I'm a navy diver, trained in pressure hulls and submarines. It was my duty to close the hatch. Had I not done this, I'm sure I would have been placed in the brig. Sir." With that, he turned and departed.

After this incident, I would leave the navy as soon as possible. I have never regretted my change of heart.

Our maker's plan was for man to be on this earth, then multiply. When I was not working on my assigned naval ship, I was doing my best to satisfy this obligation by seeking female companionship. I wasn't fussy. I was following the old, seagoing line that went: "any port in the storm," and this took me to many of the dingiest bars in lower San Diego. Here you met some of the ugliest women possible. I vividly recall one, "Twin Screw," sloppy, hooked-nosed, and sloping shoulders — a lady of the evening with a tattoo of a ship's propeller on each of her buns. With but the simplest request, she was happy to display them. Twin Screw was a knockout.

After several such encounters inside beer-stained bars on San Diego's Third Street, I began visiting local bars in the towns of Mission Beach and Ocean Beach where the pickings were of a slightly higher caliber. To my dismay, it appeared everyone could tell I was in the navy, no matter what kind of civilian clothing I wore. I might as well have had my service number tattooed on my forehead.

One mid-summer Saturday, I entered a small, older restaurant in Ocean Beach where the tables were being served by a rather thin, well-used girl, Kay. She was available, but not to me. She told me she had a boyfriend of whom she was very fond, and she let me know I was wasting my time.

Sitting in the booth behind me were two men and, I could tell by the accent, one was from Texas. The conversation was anything but humble and, as I continued to eavesdrop, I realized the Texan was talking about diving. Scuba-diving was new to the world in 1955, so chances were he was referring to abalone diving in heavy gear. "Ed," he said," I go down so darned fast I can steer with my feet." This guy was either the world's best diver, or I was hearing a story to put most attorneys to shame. I turned to get a look at him.

Both were in their late twenties and the one with the accent had a receding chin, thinning brown hair, and was wearing shorts and a loud Hawaiian shirt. His friend was smaller, with a chiseled face.

I introduced myself. "I couldn't help but overhear your conversation," I told them. "It's my guess you are abalone divers."

"Well, we sure are. I'm Todd, by God; Jerry Todd, best abalone diver on this here coast. My friend here is Nasty Ed, the nastiest man is all San Diego." Both men were wearing similar outfits, but Ed's shorts and shirt were dirtier. As a matter of fact, Ed himself was a mess.

"My name is Bob Kirby," I said, holding out a hand. "I'm a diver on a sub tender anchored in San Diego Channel."

"No kidding!" Jerry exclaimed. "I was a navy diver during the war. I'll bet I pulled up more bodies from Subic Bay than any other man. I had a wife on the beach that I traded a carton of cigarettes for. She was as ugly as could be — had a pancake face. I set her free once the war was over. Come on over here and we'll talk about diving."

I moved into their booth, and the thin waitress came over to the table. "Can I fill your cups again?" Kay was perhaps twenty-five, but heavy smoking, long working hours, and excessive drinking had cheated her of her youth. She gave me a soft smile and was much less formal than when she had first waited on me. It was easy to see Mr. Todd was the boyfriend for whom she had strong feelings. As she turned, she whisked her short skirt against Jerry's face. His conversation stopped briefly.

I learned Jerry Todd was from a small Texas town just north of Abilene. With the war, he was introduced to the ocean. His naval education led him to seek work as a civilian diver and, diving for abalone, he made good money and still had time to party. Of course I had no idea, sharing his booth that day, that Jerry would become a close friend. We ended up working together in the diving industry until he died of cancer in 1993. One thing I was assured of over those years: my friend Jerry never boasted unless it was true.

Nasty Ed had been a marine during the war, and he had earned a Purple Heart during the Iwo Jima landing. He found a bottle of sake in the bottom of a shell hole, devoured it, and passed out. His leg had been broken when he was tossed in the body cart the following morning. This, his only war wound, was the reason he was transferred back to the States. Since then he had worked hard at enhancing his chosen handle and reputation.

Nasty Ed, who was born in France, was brought to the United States as a youth, and he had retained a slight French accent. His mother was a wealthy countess, and Ed was supposed to inherit a fortune when she died. Realizing he would simply stay drunk until the money was consumed, she retained it as long as she could. She never turned a dime over to my nasty little friend, and she outlived him as well. Twenty-five years after our first meeting, Ed died on Santa Catalina Island of booze, cancer, and lead poisoning after shooting himself when his pain became unbearable. In the meantime, Ed made his mark. Every diver knew him, but nobody wanted to imitate him. The nickname, "Nasty Ed," was well-earned.

I had been warned by Jerry never to go out on the town with this foul-smelling little man because, one way or another, Ed would always end up in a fight. The one time I did not follow Jerry's advice, Ed appointed me as his stand-in – he told me he had a bad back. His back injury resulted from a boot that had been jammed under his mattress on Jerry's boat for six months. Ed was apparently too lazy to remove it. Anyway, he didn't like to fight; he enjoyed watching others fight instead. And, since I detested fighting, I followed Jerry's advice from then on.

Jerry, Ed and I left the restaurant and drove to the south side of Point Loma. Jerry wanted me to see his boat, the *Sea Deuce*, which was tied up at Carl Eychenlob's boat works. Jerry had constructed the *Sea Deuce* – so-named because it was his second boat – and he told me his first boat was called the *Sea Daddy,* a name Jerry often used in reference to himself.

The *Sea Deuce* was a modern, live-aboard boat with berths forward and an open flying bridge over the cabin. The thirty-foot craft had a cot adjacent Jerry's prized Chrysler engine. Ed slept in the forward berth while Jerry slept next to his blue power plant. The *Sea Deuce* was fast for its day, capable of making twelve or thirteen knots. The boat's operator, George Rebuck, was a large man and he stood at the controls inside the flying bridge when Jerry was diving. He also looked out over Ed who was on the bow, tending hose and cutting kelp.

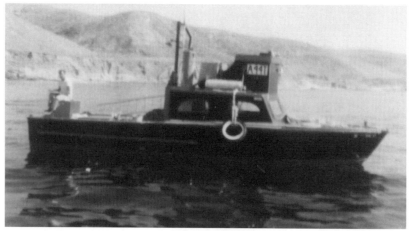

Scrap Lundy

SEA DEUCE, 1955

Their system was known as "live-boating." The boat followed the diver who was able to travel over the bottom with considerable speed. The name of the game was to cover as much bottom as possible because, by that time, the abalone were thinning out. The disadvantage of live-boating was the constant danger of the diver's hose winding up in the boat's propeller or, even worse, being cut off.

Jerry had converted a Japanese diving helmet, and it was secured to the left side of the cabin's upper deck. He had added a large faceplate and installed a water valve for air control. He did all the work himself and, while it was not beautiful, it was operational. This was Jerry's style — a bottle of Scotch and tools that were pieces of rust attached to wooden handles. Everything he owned, including the *Sea Deuce*, worked just well enough to get the job done. His simple designs were well thought out, however; the products of extensive diving experience. Several hours into our friendship, he asked me to take a one-week leave and learn to become an abalone diver. I eagerly accepted.

Processing the paperwork for my leave did not take long. By including two weekends, my five-day absence yielded nine consecutive days. Surely, nine days would be enough to educate a second-class navy diver the technique of live-boating for abalone. I had no idea my lessons would include more than diving. The fact is, I would learn nothing about being under the water at all.

When I arrived on the fishing dock, I carried my loot bag with necessary clothing including a navy-issue, woolen swimsuit. "Hi Jerry," I yelled. "I'm here."

There was no movement on the boat, and no sign of preparation for a day at sea.

Except for some strange sounds coming from below, all was quiet on board.

I stepped onto the deck and peered through the hatch into what appeared to be the remains of a party. Clothing was strewn about, not all of it belonging to a male. In the middle of the wrinkled clothing was a large, partially empty bottle of white wine – not your usual wine bottle but a five-gallon water bottle. Next to the wine sat an empty bottle of Scotch. On the cot next to his prized engine sat our skipper, wearing only what God had given him and playing a four-string banjo with one string missing. The words coming from his mouth were, perhaps, recognizable, but the sounds emitted from the old and out-of-tune instrument were not.

"Me and my wife...*plunk*...we live alone...*plunk*...in a little brown jug...*plunk*...we call our home...*plunk plunk*."

The woman occupying Ed's bunk looked, for all the world, like the waitress from the Ocean Beach cafe. She was as naked as Jerry, and she didn't move when I came down the ladder. She then, very slowly, pulled up the only blanket. "Kirby," Jerry welcomed me, "well doggone now; it's time to teach you to be an abalone diver. To begin with, I want you to meet Kay. Kay, say something to Kirby here." There was no movement, no sound.

"Well, Kirby, today our first lesson is how to buy muscatel wine." Jerry put on shorts divorced of underwear plus a badly wrinkled short-sleeved shirt, and a pair of zoris. "Come on, Kirby. We'll take my Cadillac to Escondido and buy fifteen gallons of muscadoodle."

When we arrived at the small winery, Jerry opened the large trunk of his dark blue Cadillac, revealing three empty, five-gallon water jugs. The summer Southern California desert months were living up to their reputation, and each jug was as hot as the inside of the trunk.

"Fill 'em up, Alex," Jerry said. "Now, after we get a bite to eat it's off to La Jolla Cove. We'll pack one of these bottles down to the beach, get drunk, and meet some girls. What do you think of that, Kirby?"

I had noticed the rest of Jerry's gear in the back seat – a swimsuit, a towel, baby oil, paper cups, and nothing else.

After a frightening trip down a steep, rocky trail while carrying five gallons of warm wine, we stretched out on the sand. No blankets or umbrellas; just Jerry and I with baby oil, hot wine, and soggy cups. We lay down, covered ourselves with the sticky, sweet smelly oil, and there we remained for the rest of the day, drinking hot wine until we were too sick to drink any more. The girls were everywhere and, though many knew Mr. Todd, not one gave us a second glance.

That evening we stopped at Knox Harris's house in downtown La Jolla; a clapboard beach cottage built in the thirties, small with a large yard. An enormous, cast-iron pot once used by whalers to reduce blubber sat in the middle of the yard, surrounded by driftwood.

9

Knox, a local lifeguard, had a broad smile, a winning personality, and skin the texture of brown leather. I soon learned the drill. Knox would persuade his friend Henry Hanson, a black man, to take off his swimsuit and climb into the cast-iron, water-filled pot. Then Knox would place a shiny top hat on Henry's head and someone would light the fire. Everyone would laugh, drink wine, and the party would begin. Henry climbed out before things heated up, of course. Minus his shorts. Henry was well-endowed. All the girls loved his act.

Knox and his wife had what is now referred to as an open marriage – each went his/her separate way. Many of Knox's friends were women – few of whom would get far in a beauty contest. One woman, a blonde whose hair was interwoven with strands of gray, wore a sarong wrapped only around her waist. Her breasts pointed straight down and, occasionally, she revealed her other body parts. Several of the women were wearing only short shorts or bathing suit bottoms; no tops. Nobody seemed to notice or care.

The small cottage had two bedrooms and, all evening, couples entered, did their thing, changed partners, and repeated the process. The doors were never closed and everyone appeared oblivious. We were, after all, gentle men and gentle ladies of excellent breeding.

We enjoyed lobsters for dinner – very large ones. The boiling of the beasts was part of the ceremony, for the lobsters were immersed in the pot (after Henry had climbed out, of course, and the water had reached a boil). Additional meat was prepared in a variety of ways; some was not even cooked. We ate with our bare hands, then threw the bones and carcasses into the fire. The party ended with a ceremonial, mass urination into the inferno.

Then Jerry poured me into his Cadillac and we headed back to the *Sea Deuce*. Ed was staying with a girlfriend in Mission Beach, so I slept in his bunk. (He later complained that she was a pig.)

One night Kay appeared at the boat's open hatch. "Jerry," she said, "move over."

"No Kay," he told her. "I'm tired. Go to bed in the forecastle."

"*Please...Jerry.*"

"No Kay. I'm too tired."

I began to chuckle. "You have another woman in the bow!" Kay screamed before storming off. The next day Jerry told me he thought he had a dose and hadn't wanted to tell her. He might as well have confessed, because she never dated mister Todd again.

Five days into our routine and we were still hiking down the steep trail packing a jug of hot putrid wine, laying in the warm sand, drinking our muscadoodle, and ending up totally sunburned. As a red-haired man who sunburns easily, my freckles were growing closer and closer together, and my now-stiff, navy-issue swimsuit smelled like the duty towel in a brothel. Each day ended with a wild party at Knox's, and I was beginning to wear thin.

Then Jerry laid out his new plan. We were at the beach in the cove when he said, "Kirby, today we're going to pick up a couple of girls and take them to the *Sea Deuce* for a boat ride. There's lots of wine aboard, and we'll take off our clothes and explain we're going native." He ended this plan with a wink.

"What kind of girls would even talk to two smelly, sunburned drunks like us?" I asked.

Mister Todd agreed and, with a sigh, he rolled over in the warm sand and fell fast asleep.

I awakened him an hour later. "We've been on this beach for the past seven days. All we've accomplished is getting drunk, sunburned and sick. My leave is almost over. When are you going to teach me to be an abalone diver?"

Jerry turned his sand-covered head and bloodshot eyes in my direction.

"Well now, doggone," he told me. "I already have."

The Diver

The deep sea diver is a man
Alone within his soul
His eyes and nose are full of brine
His mind is full of woe

The world he sees is dark and cold
The clammy deep his grave
There are some who say he's bold
And some may think him brave

But divers know the world below
Belongs to just a few
Who meet the challenge of the deep
With wonder ever new

G.G. Ainsworth

THE YOUNG FISH COP

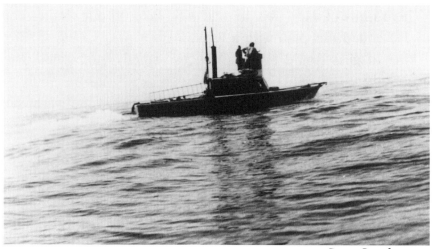

Scrap Lundy

SEA DEUCE UNDERWAY

One more evening of partying at Knox's and our days of wine, women and song would end. Tomorrow we would make it into the kelp, and I would begin my adventures as an abalone diver.

The following morning found the bow of Jerry's gray *Sea Deuce* parting the blue seas off La Jolla. My new friend was in his bunk, sleeping off a hangover. I was in little better form, having left my breakfast on the foaming waters during the short voyage.

George "Buck" Rebuck understood Jerry Todd and his wicked ways, for the two of them had worked together for several years. Rebuck's wife, Neva, a most god-fearing lady, had done her best to help Jerry "clean up his act," and convert him into a decent human being. This could be compared to teaching a pig to sing — a waste of her time and an aggravation to the pig.

Buck had long ago accepted his boss the way he was. "Well Jerry," he said, "I guess it's off to La Jolla today. I can see you didn't get to bed last night."

"Yup," Jerry answered as he hit the sack.

The one-hour run to La Jolla was enough time for our diver to recharge his batteries — to some degree at least. When Buck pulled back on the throttle, Jerry emerged. "Well," he muttered while looking around, "Guess what, Buck. It's foggy on the beach. Let's go in."

The California Department of Fish and Game required commercial divers to work in water at least twenty-feet deep in order to preserve the shallow abalone for sport divers

− commercial divers violated this rule whenever possible, of course.

A blanket of fog afforded great cover. On clear days, if someone living in an ocean-front home observed a diver working in shallow waters, he would call and turn the diver in to the fish and game. All the abalone boats were required to display large, bold numbers for identification − an aid in catching them.

This particular summer day the surf was flat, emitting little breaker noise. Jerry knew our exhaust could be heard over a mile away, a giveaway. But he also knew the fish cop on duty was a rookie who lacked experience dealing with nasty abalone divers. Messing with the fish and game wardens was one of Jerry's favorite hobbies. This would be a day when Jerry could display his love and a day our rookie warden would never forget.

Abalone are actually sea snails with a hard shell on top and a suction foot on the bottom. As a rule, they do not travel; those that do travel move very slowly. Most remain on the same rock their entire lives.

"Jerry," Buck said into the diver telephone, "you'd better come up. A fish and game boat is pulling alongside."

The young fish and game officer, dressed in perfect uniform, addressed us over his loud speaker. Because of our boat's identification number, he knew the owner. "Okay, Todd," he said, "we've caught you in shallow water. You'd better come up on deck."

"Okay, sir," Todd shouted over the noisy exhaust, "but first let me explain. We began early this morning before the sun was up. I started working this herd of abalone in deep water, but they ran like mad. I had a terrible time rounding them up as they fled into a box canyon and the protection of these shallow rocks. I guess we've been at it for three or four hours now. I know we're in shallow water, but we started out very deep. Can you see yourself clear to let us go this one time?"

The young cop agreed to the plea and even allowed us to finish our roundup in the shallow water zone before moving further offshore. His gray government boat stood by to make sure we moved out, then sped off towards San Diego.

My training continued as George put me at the controls while giving me a rundown on how to follow a diver. He was a very competent teacher; although he was slow to speak, his lecture was complete. "Keep the bubbles right there, Kirby," he told me, "right to our left. Stay back. Don't take any chances with Jerry's hose getting in the propeller." By the end of the day, I was able to control the boat in a reasonably decent manner.

Jerry had been transformed from the casual, carefree person I knew on the beach. Here in the kelp, he was all business. No time for joking; only time for hard work.

Ed cut kelp to keep the hose clear and lifted the heavy bags of abalone up and onto the deck. He measured those of questionable size, throwing back the "shorts." He was then back to the bow to tend hose.

Rebuck kept the *Sea Deuce* in position. Not once did the hose drift back. The work was intense, professional, and I was very impressed. By four o'clock, we had a good load − perhaps twenty-five-dozen big reds.

As the sun lowered, Jerry dressed out, and we were off on a good hour-and-a-half run to Eli Ready's processing plant at the fish market docks in downtown San Diego. Eli was an Oklahoma transplant. Tall and lanky, he wore cowboy boots, Levis, and a long-sleeved western shirt. I don't know how he ended up at the market because he was not suited to be a fish buyer. He was far too honest and he didn't speak Italian.

This was my introduction to Ali Baba and the Forty Thieves − the many fish markets and buyers whose businesses line up side-by-side along the San Diego waterfront. With the exception of Eli, everyone was related. Eventually, and sadly for all, this tall skinny abalone processor eventually gave up and got out. He could not overcome his ethnic background.

As Jerry had predicted, the new fish cop was waiting on the dock, and he was mad as a gaggle of Democrats caught inside a Republican convention. "Migrating abalone my ass!" he shouted. "If I ever catch you again, it'll be the slammer. Do you understand? The frigging slammer!!!"

Jerry grinned, then offered the rookie a glass of wine. "Kirby," Jerry said later when the two of us were below deck, "we got him good that time."

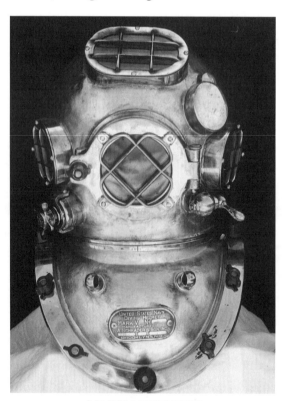

MARK V HELMET

The following day, Jerry took the time to put me down. I was not new to heavy gear, having used the Mark V helmet at Pearl Harbor's navy diving school. I hated the naval monster. It was cumbersome, restrictive, and the view port was far too small. It was my theory that Chief Stillson, the man who came up with this stupid 1915 naval design, had but one eye. The front port was much too small to accommodate both eyes at once.

This heavy gear navy training was not the first time I had been underwater wearing a copper helmet, however. When I graduated from high school in 1951, I was hired by the California Fish and Game Biology Division (not the fish cops), and we conducted a variety of fish surveys, including an abalone survey. One day at the Palo Alto office, I was introduced to Glen Bickford and "Pinky" Thomas.

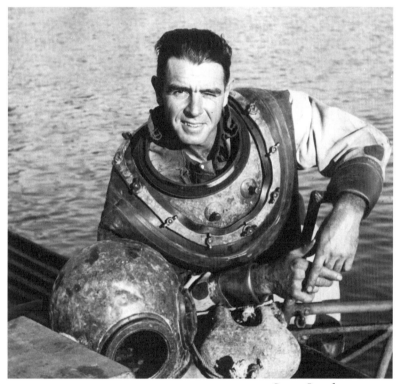

Scrap Lundy

GLEN BICKFORD

At one time Glen had been a Morro Bay abalone diver. He was dark with piercing eyes and a soft smile. In 1952 he sold his abalone boat, the *Mollusk*, to the California Fish and Game for their surveys. Pinky, a large man with a ruddy complexion, was Glen's operator, and the two of them were hired by the fish and game to run and dive the survey.

Glen winked at Pinky as he invited me to try my hand, diving at Whaler's Cove in Monterey the following Monday.

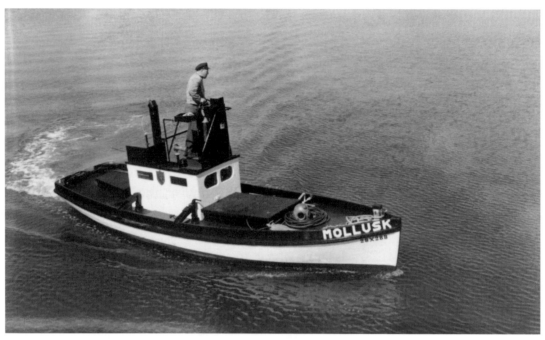

Scrap Lundy

MOLLUSK

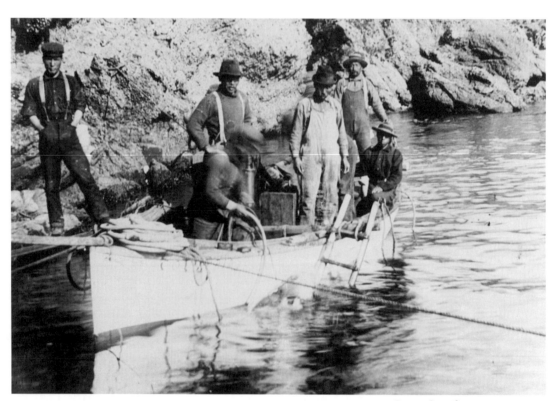

Scrap Lundy

JAPANESE DIVING BOAT

16

The abalone diving industry originated at this cove in Monterey. Here, at the turn of the century the Chinese, and later the Japanese, dove for and processed this delightful shellfish for export to their homelands. From possibly the early 1920s until World War II, the Japanese used Siino boats constructed in Monterey by Angelo Siino, an Italian boat builder. These boats were twenty-six feet in length and resembled the traditional Monterey fishing boat minus the clipper bows and semi-rounded stern. They were powered by a single sculling oar mounted onto the square stern. The diver's air compressors were hand-cranked.

In the forties these boats were outfitted with engine-powered compressors plus an engine for moving the boat around. The *Mollusk* was one of these conversions.

The Japanese diving helmet and diving dress were retained until the advent of swim gear in the fifties and sixties. This wonderful old heavy gear design was, and is, the most comfortable of all, and it is still preferred by many construction divers today.

Returning to my diving lessons in La Jolla. Jerry's helmet, although crude, was a joy to use. It had good balance and afforded visibility. As directed by Mister Todd, by constantly nudging my exhaust valve with the back of my head, I had complete control over the rig's buoyancy – a great aid in rapid movement.

The "dressing-in" procedure is much quicker than navy practice. Once the breastplate was bolted to the dress, the only items remaining were the heavy walking shoes, a leather belt holding the high-pressure bailout bottle, and the weights.

I mounted the ladder hinged to the left side of the *Sea Deuce*. As I stood there, Ed placed the helmet over my head and onto the breastplate, mating it to the interrupted threads with an eighth turn to my right. He then secured the helmet's safety latch and snapped the hose's hook to a loop onto my belt.

Two taps on the hat indicated all was ready and, as Jerry had done, I swung sideways off the ladder and into the water. Buck then backed up the boat, properly positioning it.

As a rule, the diver controls his own descent with his exhaust valve, his air inlet valve, and his posture in the water. To descend, he depresses the exhaust valve with the back of his head, releasing air from his rig. To arrest his descent, the diver opens up his air inlet valve and, bending over, traps a volume of air in the back of the dress. It took little time to master this technique. I must admit to having some trouble in this regard on my first dive, but I made it to the bottom without bursting my eardrums.

Three layers of woolen underwear would keep me warm in the sixty-degree Pacific water. If, by some fluke, the dress leaked, hypothermia would reduce my bottom time to but a portion of my normal duration.

Once on the bottom I entered a different world. I was surrounded by beautiful colors — nature's kaleidoscope. Giant green pea kelp, with its umbrella of plumage on the surface, cast ever-changing shadows on the calico ocean floor — patterns of colors moving this way and that and sea life of all descriptions. I had entered a new and enchanting place, and I almost forgot about searching for abalone.

Nevertheless, I had to make an attempt or Jerry would insist I surface and he would go down himself. Time was money. I had to locate abalone — this day's lesson in economics.

Abalone live on rocks and eat by filtering passing particles of kelp. In order to survive, they must inhabit an environment of cool, moving, unpolluted water. Baby abalone grow under rocks, some remain in one spot their entire lives. Others may migrate, often selecting an upside-down life under rock shelves. These are the most difficult to spot; their small black tentacles give them away.

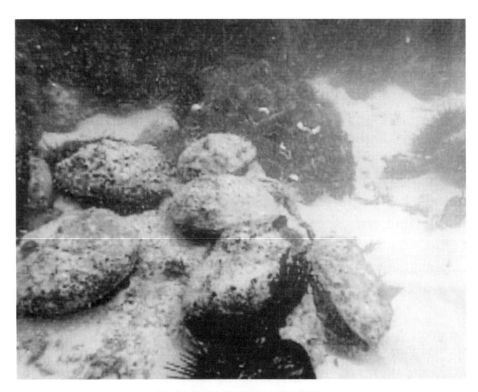

ABALONE UNDER WATER

Moving on the bottom in heavy gear is much like climbing a sand dune, and the toes of the metal boots are used for traction. I had to work hard to cover ground quickly, laying over at a forty-five-degree angle to the bottom due to the adverse forces constantly pulling on me. The surge can be severe — it has been known to run a diver twenty feet in both directions. Because there is a constant danger of being forced into a rock and smashing the glass, most abalone helmets have been refitted with very strong plastic ports.

An abalone bar is used to pry, and then break, the suction the abalone has on the rock. It is also used to cut kelp in the path of the diver's hose and to measure the abalone.

The net bag has a one-foot-diameter ring attached to its top through which the abalone are placed. Once the bag is full, the tender throws a weighted bag line, with an empty bag attached, to the diver's bubbles. It usually falls close. The diver then unsnaps the empty and snaps on a full bag. Once I had filled my bag − a task that took me much longer than it had taken Jerry − I was asked to come up and Jerry took my place. I then resumed my boat-operating lessons.

After years of reflection, I realized this day was one of great significance. While the diving education was a very necessary stepping stone in my life, my lessons with George Rebuck turned out to be the most important. I not only learned how to operate a boat; I also learned how to educate others, a skill which served me when I became an instructor at Santa Barbara City College in 1982.

What did I teach? A host of subjects including how to operate a boat. George Rebuck, who had been patient with me as a teacher, was my mentor and I tried to follow his example.

Last of all, this was the day Jerry and I signed a pact in blood. From this day on, we would do anything that caused unpleasantness for the fish cops.

In 1999, using real shells, I constructed a dozen fake abalones. The meat was composed of automotive body filler and the tentacles were made from inner tubes. I used black bathtub caulking as the soft meat around the base of the shell, and my fake abalones looked very real.

By a stroke of luck, Scrap Lundy, author of *The California Abalone Industry*, and I were hired by Huell Houser, producer of the popular TV series "California's Gold," to assist him in filming the oldest, still-surviving, Japanese diver plus highlights of the now-defunct abalone industry. We rented an old wooden fishing boat, and the filming took place in the waters off the Monterey Aquarium where we were surrounded by kelp and sea otters. No abalone had been seen in the area for over forty years; something any fish cop should have known.

During the shoot a gray fish and game boat approached, moving at top speed and spraying water everywhere. "What are you doing?" the warden shouted through his speaker. I held up one of my fake large reds and shook it at him. "Drop that abalone," he yelled, eyes wild.

"Why would I want to drop it?" I asked. "These are very expensive. I'm not going to drop it."

He went for his gun. During this entire encounter his boat was continually drifting, and it finally ended up against our old Monterey fishing boat. We had a ranger aboard, Jerry Loomis from Point Lobos, and he addressed the warden. "John," he said, "this is a fake abalone. Take it and look it over."

The warden checked it out, then returned it with an "Okay. I'll let you go this time."

What a jerk.

"John," I yelled as the warden departed. "I just want you to have a nice day." Our tax dollars at work.

Someday I'll be joining Jerry Todd up there. We'll be together again, recalling this incident and laughing our wings off.

I doubt if Warden John will be joining us, however.

My future was mandated with Jerry Todd's heavy gear lessons on the *Sea Deuce*. I would be a commercial diver or, at the very least, I would be involved in diving for the rest of my life. It seems strange to me now, however, that this lifelong vocation was the result of pure chance. I was in the right place at the right time, drinking coffee in a restaurant. If I hadn't met Mister Todd, it is difficult to say where or what I would be doing today.

The following weekend I once again left my naval ship and headed for the *Sea Deuce*. I glanced into the boat's engine room and berth area. Everything was shipshape, ready for work. Mister Todd had stopped partying. I anticipated spending the next two days watching my talented friend move over the ocean floor like one of George Patton's tanks.

Jerry did not want to be slowed down this day, and I tended and operated with Buck at my side. My diving lessons would have to wait until another time. At our short noon break we tied alongside the *Mable*, a small boat owned by Lad Handelman and Rex Rosenberry. Lad, a rather small man, was on deck tending – Rex was diving. The irritating clatter of their single-cylinder compressor destroyed the peaceful environment, and the insane racket echoed back at us from the shear, Point Loma cliffs, doubling the noise. Once Rex surfaced, the compressor could be silenced. I vowed never to own such a monster; a mistake that would try my future marriage and, at the same time, come close to ending my life.

The *Mable*, a smaller and older boat than the *Sea Deuce*, was tied to the surface kelp instead of being anchored or live-boated. Three hundred feet of diving hose was then played over her weathered rail.

Lad and Rex were "dead-boating"; instead of following the diver, the boat was anchored. In order for the diver to cover as much bottom as possible at a single anchoring, the long hose was necessary.

Instead of heavy gear, they employed swim gear – mask, dry suit, and weights. Lad and Rex walked on the bottom; most other dead-boaters swam, using fins and a lighter weight belt.

Rex signaled Lad to take up his slack. He was coming up. Through an eruption of bubbles, a tall and very cold man appeared. He removed his mask and replaced his glasses (this was half a century before today's lasic surgery). Rex couldn't wear his thick glasses within the frame of the aluminum mask. Blind as a bat, he had to go without.

Rex and Lad shared a strange partnership. Lad was a handsome and very determined seventeen-year-old who could easily run through the kelp and rocks, quickly filling one bag and returning for an empty. He could gather ten dozen abalone in half a day − almost as many as Jerry Todd could gather in that length of time. On the other hand, because of his poor vision, Rex had to feel his way through the rocks. He moved so slowly that his body couldn't heat up. He always came up cold and with very few abalones − sometimes none − and, on more than one occasion, he was carrying a rock that he thought was a mollusk.

In Lad and Rex's favor, the twenty-five-foot *Mable* was inexpensive to own and operate and only had to support two crew members. Still, their harvest was seldom adequate.

Lad had a very strong sense of loyalty which was to serve him well in later years, for he was to eventually found and control Oceaneering, the world's largest diving company. He could never ask Rex to quit; however, something had to change.

In an effort to assist, Nasty Ed announced he might go aboard the *Mable* as a diver. Rex could remain on deck and tend Lad and Ed at the same time. All three would share their proceeds equally.

The evening run to Eli Ready's was rather somber. Jerry had to decide between finding another tender in San Diego or moving to Morro Bay and joining Barney Clancy's famous Black Fleet. The following morning, Jerry announced they would load the *Sea Deuce* with as many items as possible and head north. George Rebuck would also move his family to Morro Bay while Nasty Ed would move in with Rex and Lad who were living in Ocean Beach.

One problem remained. George had to sell the *Laura Belle,* the boat he had built to fish both albacore and swordfish. I volunteered to babysit her until George could find a buyer. She was a handsome vessel and would make a fine temporary home for me while providing a possible second income. George allowed me to equip her with a compressor for dead-boating.

I asked if I might also dive and tend on the *Mable*. I agreed to help with the problems on this aging craft by using the mechanical experience and resources I had gained in the navy. I considered all this to be a piece of cake. I decided I might even attempt to design and construct an improved, wider diving mask. The cast-aluminum Widoff was far too narrow to fit my fat face and, by the end of one hour on the bottom, I felt as if my cheeks had been reshaped by an hydraulic press.

The USS *Nereus* housed every kind of shop known − machine shop, welding shop, dive locker, and foundry plus a host of other facilities. Designing and constructing masks and related diving equipment would be simple, or so it seemed to me at the time. I intended to copy a mask of stainless steel sheet metal that Henry Hanson made. Hanson, the man in the pot at Knox's party, was a welder in the naval shipyard, and he had built several masks for friends and for his own weekend use.

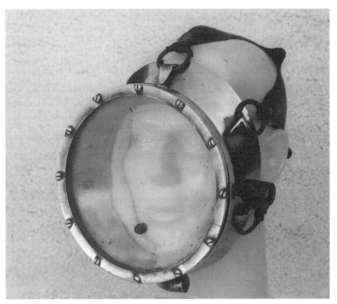

KIRBY #1 MASK PROTOTYPE — MADE ON THE *NEREUS*, 1955

After I built the prototype (which I still have) I set out to build ten more — a small production line funded by Uncle Sam. I figured that when my ship went to sea, I could continue working in the abalone industry right in the ship's shop. Chief Haney came completely unglued. "These things aren't navy-approved!" Undaunted, I continued with my masks — the first in the Kirby line of diving equipment.

I spent a lot of time with Lad, Rex and Ed at their Ocean Beach house, where Lad's mother had recently moved in. Every evening was consumed with conversations concerning abalone, the making of bags, and the repairing of many leaks in their Belle Aqua dry suits.

One night Lad told me the sad story of his introduction to diving the previous year. His uncle, Jimmy Pirog, was a former prize fighter, and he had a bad temper. Sometime toward the decade that ended WWII, Jimmy had moved to Los Angeles from Philadelphia to attend the Sparling School of Diving and Underwater Welding in Wilmington. After graduating he started a short-lived partnership with a fellow graduate, Whitey Stefens. They bought a fantailed fishing boat, the *Sylvia J*, and outfitted her for abalone live-boating.

Unfortunately, due to Jimmy's temper and lack of human understanding, plus sloppy unseaworthy workmanship and equipment, the partnership failed. According to Lad, a four-day trip to San Clemente Island would be spent in total silence because a single word by Lad or Whitey might cause Jimmy to go ballistic and a fist fight would follow.

After the breakup, Jimmy bought out Whitey and moved the *Sylvia J* to San Diego.

Here he had met Jerry Todd who soon became a close friend — at sea, Jimmy was a tyrant but, on the beach, he could be a great person.

The *Sylvia J* had not seen fresh paint since the partnership had dissolved. The compressor was so rusty it was unrecognizable and, after its mounting bracket had rusted away, the fuel tank was hung from the mast with rope.

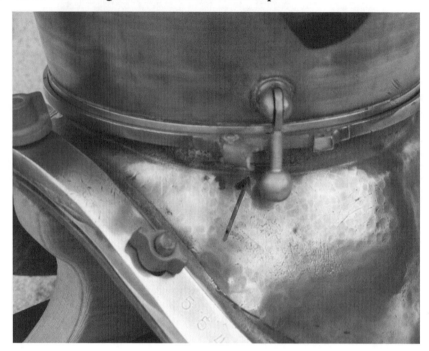

BROKEN HELMET LATCH

Jimmy used a USN Mark V helmet that was minus the safety catch, a device that prevented the hat from coming unscrewed. The old Mark V was fitted with an air control valve divorced of its handle, and Jimmy had wired a pair of pliers to the helmet, a tool with which to open and close this valve. Using thick plexiglas, he had installed a larger view port, but with rusting steel hardware. Every other piece of his gear, including the *Sylvia J* itself, was on the verge of falling apart.

Successful commercial fishing requires regular maintenance of equipment plus a few, clever innovations. Fishermen who are unsuccessful have usually violated this formula. It was inevitable that Jimmy Pirog would fail; the question was simply — when? His love of women and partying overshadowed any type of maintenance, as he simply did not have time to work on his old boat.

At Jimmy's invitation, Lad had come out to California from the Bronx. Like his fierce uncle, Lad had been raised with his fists. He was a tough young man who didn't know how to back down. He knew a lot about people but nothing about machinery — there was no room for mechanical toys in his childhood. He had never driven a car, nor had he worked on one. He never thought about nuts and bolts, only about how to get along with others and how to win. Winning with honor was Lad's life. It didn't matter how difficult the task — one way or the other, he would prevail.

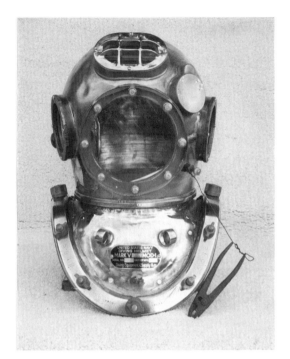 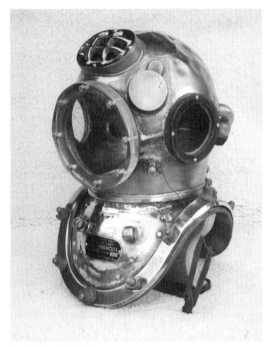

PIROG'S HELMET

He could not endure his bad-tempered uncle, however, and after sticking it out for a month, he ended up picking lemons in Orange County. Anything was better than working with Pirog.

Pirog would occasionally entice a tourist to come onboard for a look at his operation, and he would then offer to take the gentleman for a short ride around the harbor. This ride could turn into a one-week trip to San Clemente Island, sixty miles northwest of San Diego. When the now-alert visitor began to protest and carry on, Jimmy would tell him to jump off and swim for it. Good grief. Jimmy Pirog was a real bastard.

The moment his helmet was removed, Pirog would demand a lighted cigarette be placed in his mouth. Once when A.J. Grubb, his operator, was thirty seconds late with the cigarette, Pirog had Lad remove his entire outfit, then he ran the *Sylvia J* up against a rock and ordered A.J. off the boat. Grubb broke down, begging forgiveness. Next time, he had a lighted cigarette ready. I've heard that Jimmy Pirog actually put one tender off on a rock and left him there. Had it not been for a passing boat, the man would have perished.

Pirog had such a deadly temper that you could be taking your life in your hands, bringing him up from a dive in an emergency. Eventually, no man — whether shanghaied or not — would work with him. Swimming ashore was better than slugging it out with Jimmy Pirog.

Once in the summer of 1955, Pirog's crew saw him climb his hose, then descend again. He often did this to clear his ears, and they knew that pulling him up to check on him was a dangerous idea. Finally, after ten minutes had passed, A.J. ordered the tender to bring Pirog to the surface. There was no point in lighting his cigarette this time — his helmet had long since come off. His dress was filled with water and it was impossible to bring his body aboard. The crew had to run back into the commercial harbor with Pirog tied to the diving ladder.

The weather-beaten *Sylvia J* was tied to a dock until Lad returned but, due to her forlorn condition, she was more of a burden to him than a profitable inheritance.

Jimmy Pirog had died several months before I met Jerry, but Jerry still had a hard time talking about it. He and Pirog had exchanged words concerning the poor condition of Pirog's equipment, and Jerry was unable to shake the feeling that he was, in some way, responsible for Pirog's death.

This death provoked many of those in the abalone fleet to reassess, and then overhaul, their gear. Some was as shoddy as Pirog's.

All this took place almost fifty years ago, and Lad had been searching all this time for his uncle's lost helmet. He managed to locate one diving shoe, but this was his only link to his deceased mentor.

Then, one day in the summer of 2000, I was browsing through an antique store in Ventura when I spotted a beat-up old Mark V sitting on a top shelf. I recalled the helmet from my days with Associated Divers in 1964. Jerry Todd had owned it and he brought it into our shop one day and asked me to cut it up. "Kirby," he insisted, "remove any useful parts and get rid of the rest." Jerry loved everyone and hung onto everything, so this was out of character for him. I wondered why he was so upset with an old navy hat. This question remained unresolved until I saw the remainder of the Mark V in the antique store.

Jerry had taken Pirog's helmet off the *Sylvia J* and had stored it until the days of Associated Divers. He had asked me to cut it up as a parting farewell to his former friend. When Associated Diver's went out of business, what was left of the old hat was purchased along with a lot of other crap. How ironic that it should show up years later and, even more ironic, that I should be the one to discover it — the one person in the world who knew the whole story.

I phoned Phil Nuytten, and he offered to send me $500 to purchase the helmet. I then took it home for evaluation. Many parts were missing, but a phone call to Rick at Desco solved that, for Rick offered me all the missing parts for nothing, as a tribute to Lad Handelman.

I rebuilt the helmet, and it eventually looked about the same as it had during Pirog's last days. About this time the Historical Diving Society was hosting a symposium at Santa Barbara's new Maritime Museum, and Phil and I were allowed to give a short speech. We presented the helmet to Lad, cold turkey.

I had pictured Lad grinning from ear to ear, beside himself with pleasure while holding his Uncle Jimmy's hat in his arms. Instead, he simply sat in his wheelchair and wept. It was apparently too much for him to comprehend. Two days later, after the trauma had subsided, I told him the entire story and how I had discovered the hat.

Jimmy Pirog's helmet is sitting on Lad's living room table today, and he tells me that, when he's alone, he can hold it and talk to his uncle. I know what he means because I was aware of Pirog's presence while putting the finishing touches on his rebuilt helmet. Then the fierce little fighter was gone again.

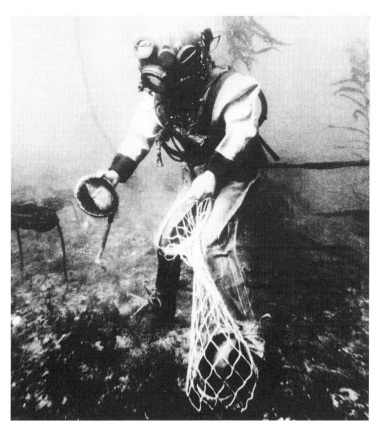

PIROG IN NAVY MARK V

27

THE *LAURA BELLE*

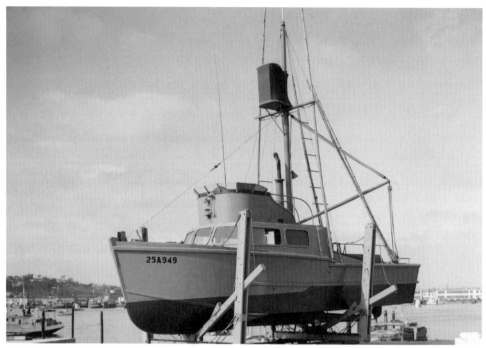

LABEL: Steve Rebuck

LAURA BELLE

I stood on the dock in San Diego's commercial harbor and watched as Jerry Todd and George Rebuck finished loading the *Sea Deuce*. George started the engine, and I waved them off, tears and all. Very soon, fond memories and the wake of Jerry's boat would be all that remained. I had found new friends in Lad and Rex, however, and I knew the year 1956 would be as exciting as those preceding it — just different.

I moved the *Laura Belle* to Jerry's empty berth at Carl Eychenlob's boat works. On the other side of the dock was a small Monterey, the *Antone*, owned by Tony Metson, an aging Greek fisherman whose once-black hair was now silver. A spirited youth, little of his original ambition remained, and most of his day was spent sitting on the *Antone's* fish hatch talking to the other fishermen. Within a short time, Tony adopted me, replacing my grandfather who had died three years earlier.

The *Antone*, once the pride of the San Diego fishing fleet, was no longer a spotless, light blue and gray, thirty-foot albacore boat. Instead, it was a muddled combination of browns — a mixture of grease, oil, and rust. Tony's out-of-tune, gasoline cook stove, mounted in the small fo'c'sle, was responsible for the soot covering everything, including the ship's master. Tony's eyes, bright as the day he was born seventy-three years earlier, were the only things reflecting light.

My occasional days at sea with Lad and Rex yielded enough extra abalone and fish to supply my old friend with seafood. Tony was a chef extraordinaire. He could take almost anything and turn it into a meal fit for a king. One day he offered to make octopus cioppino for me and serve it with Carlo Rossi paisano and French bread. "Eata the bread and drink the wine," he told me, "or your meal won't digest."

Taking his advice to heart, I made a pig of myself. Unfortunately, I was not aware that the eight-legged serpent had been laying on the deck of the *Antone* for five summer days, and that night I was as sick as it is possible to be without actually dying. The following day, I staggered over to the small albacore boat; Tony was none the worse. I learned two lessons that day − I'm not Greek and I don't have a cast-iron stomach.

One evening, sitting on the deck of the *Antone* with wine in hand, our conversation turned to swordfishing, which is gentlemen fishing in the heat of the day. This sounded like a delightful adventure − no rising at four to don clammy woolens or freeze the fingers letting out cold, wet lines when long-lining. Why not rig the *Laura Belle* for swordfish instead of abalone? At least, for awhile. Rebuck had the necessary hardware stored in the boat works, and Tony could fill me in on the details. It sounded easy. Anyway, what was there to learn?

George Rebuck, being a frugal man, had successfully converted the *Laura Belle* from a surplus, World War II landing craft, and she was well-designed. George, a soft-spoken, large man, had pinched her square bow into a fine, thin prow, and he had replaced her pointed stern with a beautifully contoured transom. Her decks were clean, a necessary requirement for swordfishing, and her large hold could accommodate five tons.

Her low pilothouse was well thought-out, with a nice galley and three berths. Her windows and overall lines showed a northern influence, and she was painted a tasteful combination of grays and whites, trimmed in black. The *Laura Belle* was a far cry from most of her southern cousins − some of the world's ugliest plywood monstrosities.

She had only one weakness, and it was a major one. In his efforts to save money, George had installed a surplus World War II tank engine, an eight-cylinder flathead Cadillac. This engine came with a devil-inspired automatic transmission. The contraption would pass through three forward gears so fast you couldn't tell them apart. This wasn't a problem but, in reverse, instead of the one-to-one final ratio she had while in forward, she had a twelve-to-one ratio. Since I could not run the engine at twelve times its proper speed, the landing craft had almost no reverse.

It took me a long time to master her. I could turn the little craft faster than I could stop her, and long range planning was the key. I had to allow time for the propeller shaft

29

brake to tighten before the reversing gears would engage. This consumed valuable seconds. The vacuum cylinder would hiss and the solenoids would snap in proper order before the propeller shaft began its slow, reverse rotation. This resulted in white-knuckled hands and heavy perspiration, all leading to heart-stopping panic everytime we docked in a marina.

Occasionally, always when yachts were nearby, the shaft brake failed. When this happened, the swearing began – first by others and then by me. The yachts' skippers were never understanding. Yachts and commercial fishing boats don't mix.

Boats rigged for swordfishing had a forward plank as long as the length of the boat. This extended over the bow like a long bowsprit on a sailboat. On the end was a pulpit, a steel basket resembling a Roman chariot. A man standing within this unstable contraption attempted to stick a harpoon through a sunning swordfish. These enormous critters, some weighing as much as five-hundred pounds, are not stupid. They weren't simply laying there, waiting to be stuck; instead, they were taking advantage of the warm middle-of-the-day sun, and they were very much awake.

To reduce the noise of the bow pounding over the waves, the boat must be stealthily maneuvered from downwind. If the fish detected pounding, it was gone in a heartbeat. When extended over a large swordfish, a skilled harpoonist is a necessity, and the boat operator must be motivated. Still, the intended victim escaped much of the time.

Outfitting the *Laura Belle* for "stick fishing" took about three weeks. I rigged our long plank which was guyed with many wires to the mast and the boat's hull. After arranging another five-day leave, I talked my shipmate and boss, Ed Lawler, into taking leave with me. As I stated earlier, Ed was a first-class shipfitter and diver and one of my closest navy friends.

The following morning the two of us sat in the flying bridge as the Cadillac's eight-cylinder engine created an even, muffled sound – soft enough to lull us to sleep. The sharp gray bow of the *Laura Belle* cut through the green waters of the channel in silence. This particular day, the often-turbulent sea was flat as a millpond.

This was the first time the two of us had commanded a small craft twelve miles offshore. We would be far beyond sight of Point Loma with its visible, high white cliffs and lighthouse that provided bright light. We had no radio, fathometer, or modern GPS – just a compass and watch. If we were fogged out, we would have to rely on our dead-reckoning skills to make it back to a safe anchorage. (As Tony once wisely told me after drinking too much paisano, "Kooby, sometimes you just gotta rely on dog-barking navigation. If you can hear the dogs barking, you are too close to the beach.")

Neither Ed nor I had ever seen a swordfish. Tony had informed us they "finned," which meant both the dorsal fin and tail would be exposed above the surface and easy to spot in a flat sea. There were only two problems – shark and marlin also finned.

Marlin are not a market fish, so they are ignored by commercial fishermen. They are fierce fighting critters, however, so they are sought after and prized by sport fishermen. Broadbill swordfish, the fish we were after, were similar in appearance but much chunkier. They also have slightly wider fins and a long sword that can be compared to the "spike" of the marlin. Consequently, it was hard for a couple of novices like us to tell the difference.

We were surrounded by sport fishing yachts with cigar-smoking owners holding rods and reels while bikini-clad girls sunned on the sterns. Our tiny work boat looked like a piece of gray waste, drifting in nature's magnificent punch bowl.

"Kirby, over there!" Ed had spotted fins and my adrenaline ran wild. "You head out the plank," I told him, "I'll take the boat upwind and make a run!" Once upwind, I turned and headed straight down onto our sunning asset. The harpoon was in Ed's hand, fire and determination were in his eyes.

A swordfish harpoon is an approximately eight-foot-long, wooden shaft with a small-diameter, flexible steel rod, referred to as a "lily iron," extending two feet from its tip. Fixed to the end of the iron is a brass dart with six hundred feet of attached manila line. This line is secured with clothespins along the bottom of the plank, then coiled into a large basket. The line's bitter end is joined to a rubber buoy, capable of supporting two-hundred pounds. Another line leads from the rubber buoy to a high spar float with a red flag.

A second, twenty-foot line secures the back end of the harpoon shaft to the pulpit's rail. Once over his target, the harpoon man does his best to shove the dart clear through the fish. If he succeeds, the fish sounds, the short line comes taut, and the dart is pulled free of the lily iron. The harpoon is then retrieved.

Ed struck hard and scored. The huge gray shape sounded for the entire six hundred feet and kept on going. The rubber buoy went over the side in a heartbeat, followed by the spar and flag. Everything stayed under water for a good ten minutes; finally the buoy, and then the flag, surfaced. Tony had warned us to wait thirty minutes to allow sea pressure to kill the fish before pulling it on board.

Ed pulled as I coiled the line back into the basket. Our prize was soon alongside, and it appeared to be about nine feet long. By this time, several sport fishing boats were circling, all eager to get a look at a broadbill.

We rigged the boat's boom over the side, secured a rope choker around the fish's tail, and strained hard on the line in an effort to haul the beast to landing height. Once clear of the rail, we swung the fish to the center of the deck where it was highly visible. Our treasure hung from the rigging where it swayed back and forth with each roll of the *Laura Belle*. It represented enough cash to finance several more days of fishing. We could purchase ice for our hold, fuel for our engine, and paisano for our bellies. Things were looking good.

Taking a breather, we noticed the crews in the surrounding boats seemed upset..*very* upset. One skipper extended his middle finger to express his mood; others cursed and tossed well-chewed cigars in the water in rage.

Ed's blonde hair was blowing in the breeze as he looked at me, his very perplexed skipper. "Kirby, is there a chance this is a marlin?" Then, "Oh my God! Quick! Ed, drop the critter on deck! I'll put wet gunny sacks over it and we'll get out of here."

Once clear of the fleet, we cleaned the enormous fish and headed back to the boat works where I gave some of the meat to anyone who would take it. Tony was our prime prospect. "Kooby," he scolded. "You're a screw-up. Don't you know the difference between a broadbill and a marlin?" The words he actually used were more colorful than those I can print. And his wrinkled face and pinched eyebrows said it with much more authority.

The following day had to be better. Much better. Ed and I headed off for the ice docks to fill our hold. I had measured the hold − simple math − and now I measured a block of ice. "Shoot me fifteen blocks," I told the black-toothed man who was operating the dock's grinder. I positioned the large diameter rubber hose into the hold's rear, kneeling down to do so. "Okay," I said, "let her rip."

"Kurump!" The first block went into the machine. The six-inch-diameter hose grew stiff and started to jump as the sharp steel impeller ground up the huge frozen mass before blowing it into our hold.

What a beautiful sight. The ice particles gleamed in the sunlight. I could envision several broadbills, all iced down and ready to market. God, how I loved this moment and this life − the life of a fisherman.

"Kurump!" A second block. The onslaught could be compared to a Tibetan avalanche as the hose once again grew stiff and bounced about as more of the valuable ice was blown into our hold. However, I was a bit confused because it seemed as if our compartment might be filling faster than I had anticipated.

"Kurump!" I suddenly realized the ice was expanding three or four times when crushed and blown. The small hold was filling so fast I might be buried.

"Kurump!" Four blocks! The frigging hold was full. I crawled out onto the deck, still holding the leaping, six-inch rubber monster.

I yelled at Ed to stop the guy, but he couldn't get up on the dock or be heard over the grinder's racket. *"Kurump!"* More freezing ice shot out of the end − a white mound piled up against the back of the boat's wheelhouse.

"Kurump!" The mound was growing fast.

"STOP THE DAMNED ICE!!"

"Kurump!" Another block of ice we didn't want and couldn't afford. (My navy pay was $100 a month; each block cost us five bucks which equated to one-day-and-a-half inside the repair shop on the USS *Nereus*, welding this and that while answering "Yes sir," whenever I was addressed. Oh well, everything in this world is relative.)

The frozen crap kept coming, one block of ice after another. I realized what was going on — the jerk with the black teeth was playing with us. There was no way a thirty-five-foot boat could use fifteen blocks of ice. He knew this and was taking advantage of our ignorance while enjoying every minute of it. Grinning from ear to ear, the bastard was pretending not to hear our shouts.

Very soon, the aft deck of the *Laura Belle* resembled an enormous ski mogul. To keep our craft from capsizing, I turned the devil-inspired hose into the water and watched as our working capital dissolved to the accompaniment of more *"Karumps!"* Fifteen in all.

Our hold filled with ice came back to haunt us the next night. It is a wonder our little fishing boat survived. I guess God loved her.

Our success at sticking a fish, even if it was the wrong breed, filled us with optimism. The following morning our youthful enthusiasm and excellent eyesight paid off. This time it was a broadbill and we got him. Before we could bring him to the surface, we stuck another. By two in the afternoon we had them both cleaned and iced.

We were alarmed at how fast our ice was disappearing while our bilges were filling up with melted water. Still, we were encouraged by the two large fish averaging 350 pounds each. At fifty cents a pound, we would soon be sharing $350, enough for gasoline, ice, and another jug of wine. Tony would be proud.

Because the day was young, instead of heading back to the boat works, we decided to run into Mission Bay, three miles north of Point Loma. We might even anchor and go ashore for a cool one...perhaps two. We were preparing to anchor when I spotted a boat also rigged for broadbill and as we approached, without mentioning our two broadbill, I did my best to start a conversation. "Hi there," I said. "We're wondering where and how to sell our fish, if we ever catch any."

"Well son," the skipper (who was quite old, perhaps forty), "that's for me to know and you to find out."

After anchoring, we rowed our skiff to the Cove Bar on the Mission Beach isthmus. Seated there, we attempted to impress a couple of single ladies by telling them we were seasoned fishermen with a fine craft at anchor, just offshore the bar.

Two additional beers cemented our plans for the evening. Darby, olive-skinned, of French descent and very attractive, would have dinner with Ed. The other, a knockout with short curly red hair, refused to divulge her name, but she agreed to return with me to the

Laura Belle for some paisano. (I was too cheap to offer dinner.)

I did my best to talk my new friend, "Red," into going for a swim with me, but she refused. She said she had promised herself to her boyfriend in baseball camp and, though I told her I understood, I spent the entire evening trying to talk her out of that plan — unsuccessfully.

Soon it was eleven and Red wanted to return to shore. She was worried about Darby; I was concerned that Ed might be freezing somewhere on the beach. As we began moving about, the *Laura Belle* took a giant roll to starboard. The roll was accompanied by a loud, crushing noise, and my feet were suddenly covered with water. My thoughts ran wild as I poked my head through the companionway. There, to my amazement, stood Ed, fully clothed and with muddy feet.

"How did you get here?" I asked.

After a difference of opinion, Ed and olive-skinned Darby had gone their separate ways. Ed had waited three hours for the tide to ebb so he could walk out to the boat. It was a moonlit night, and I could now see that we were surrounded by abandoned tires punctuated by cans, fifty-gallon oil drums, and trash. We were anchored in the middle of a marine garbage dump.

After the tide went out the *Laura Belle* had been left behind, balanced on her keel, and Ed had upset her when he climbed aboard. The boat then rolled onto its chine. The water I was standing in was ice melt, not seawater. That was good news.

The last I saw of Red was the back of her head as she walked home, with feet undoubtedly as muddy as Ed's.

Ed and I attempted to sleep in our now thirty-degree-inclined bunks as we waited for the tide to rise. It was a wonder we could sleep at all; we later discovered something buried in the undersea junk pile had stove in one of the *Laura Belle's* planks. This was the crunching sound we had heard.

Two more days of fishing resulted in two more broadbill. We were now down to the last of our ice, so we were off to Ali Baba and the Forty Thieves to convert our hold filled with cleaned fish into much-needed cash. Seven or eight fish buyers were lined up on the dock like rug merchants in a bazaar and, if they were not related, they were certainly in cahoots.

We tied up and I began negotiating with one. "How much are you paying for broadbill?" I asked.

"Son," he replied, "before I answer, climb up here. I want you to look in my refrigerator." Inside, I saw at least ten swordfish, stacked like cordwood. "See?" he continued. "I don't need your fish. I can't get rid of what I have. I'll give you twenty-seven cents a pound. That's it."

The other buyers made the same offer. We had no choice but to accept their twenty-seven cents a pound, which was half what we expected — hardly worth our effort. At the fuel dock later, we ran into the skipper of the swordfish boat — the one we had talked to earlier in the Mission Bay anchorage. When we told him about the thieves in San Diego, he was livid. "You bastard! You broke our holdout for fifty cents a pound! For two cents, I could pound your pointed head through your plywood deck!!"

I was twenty-two, rather strong, very much at home in the water, and I possessed a redhead's temper. Although I had never been much of a fighter, I wanted to get him into the water, drown him, and tie his worthless body to his own propeller. He may have sensed this because he quietly pulled away and out of Ed and my lives.

Ed was on duty the following weekend, and I didn't have enough money for fuel or ice so, seeking excitement and relaxation, I took the *Laura Belle* for a slow joy ride around the commercial harbor. It was just what the doctor ordered, me and the little swordfish boat, sailing around the harbor in the middle of the day.

As I passed the last marina, I noticed a movie company filming a commercial on an extended dock and, just for the fun of it, I decided to bring my boat in for a closer look. Considering her limited ability to back down, it would be a tight spot. "Oh well," I told myself, "I can always turn her if I get in trouble." I had completely overlooked the long plank extending over the bow.

The film crew was lined up with the cameraman in the middle; his camera on a tripod. "Action!" the director called. With this, the entire crew went into action. That same instant I realized I was too close and had run out of room in which to turn, so I hit the shaft brake button which would enable me to shift into reverse. I anxiously awaited the snap of the solenoid and the hiss of the vacuum cylinder. *Silence.* The frigging brake had failed again.

Quickly swinging the wheel hard over, I opened the throttle in an effort to come around fast enough to miss those on the dock. I was too late. The plank's pulpit and bobstay resembled a horizontal, wire guillotine, sweeping away anything standing on the dock. The crew ducked, somehow missing decapitation, and though the cameraman managed to catch his camera before it went into the drink, it was somewhat smashed. At least it didn't take a swim.

The director was furious. "You idiot. Why the hell are you in here!"

I had to think fast. "Excuse me, sir," I hollered down from the flying bridge. "Can you tell me where the fuel dock is?"

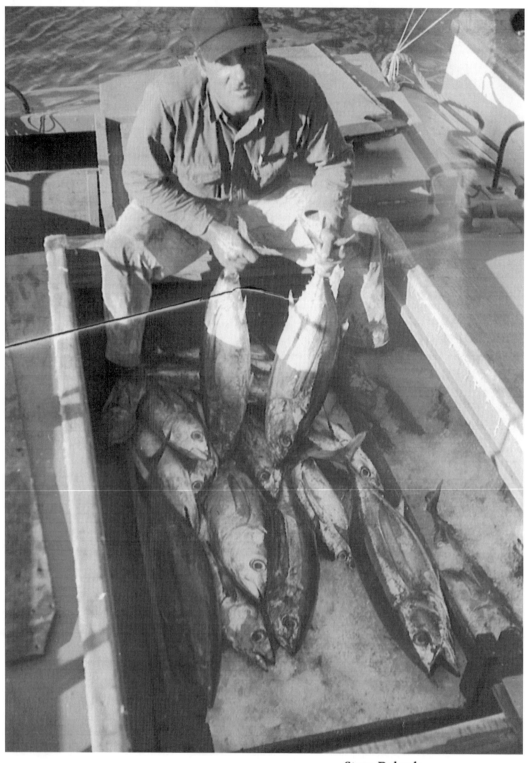

Steve Rebuck

GEORGE REBUCK, 1953

36

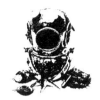

THE *RESTLESS* AND THE BOAT WORKS

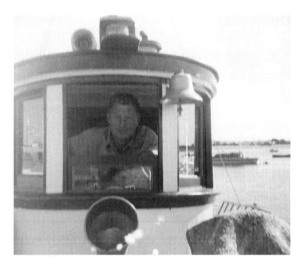

BOB STEERING THE *RESTLESS*, SAN DIEGO, 1956

Eychenlob's boat works held an assortment of floating docks in varying condition, from new to sinking, arranged in a giant U shape. The newer and most active fishing boats were tied to the newer docks; the older boats – those not in use or about to sink – were tied to the older, waterlogged docks. The only houseboat ended up in whatever space was available. I had inherited the outside dock from Jerry Todd, and it answered my need for a facility that could hold a craft of questionable maneuverability, the *Laura Belle*.

Tied to one of the sinking finger docks was the *Restless*, a small, thirty-foot, fantail trawler. Her lines were beautiful but her condition was not. She was for sale to anyone who met stringent qualifications – the applicant had to be alive and breathing.

I had just received a letter from George Rebuck telling me the new owner of the *Laura Belle* would arrive the following weekend. I would have to evacuate her, so I contacted the gentleman who owned the little trawler and struck a deal. "Six hundred bucks, as is, where is, to be paid someday." This sounded good at the time but, looking back, I should have had doubts.

The *Restless* was designed to fish albacore and had fine northern features. She had a rounded pilothouse with classic, drop-down windows, and because her fo'c'sle was of the raised-deck style, she was quite roomy for her length. Except for a fish hatch and a salmon steering hatch, her afterdeck was flush.

With her sleek hull, she could slip through the water with ease. Consequently, she required only a small engine for power. This gave her a long range. From a distance she appeared to be forty or fifty feet long. However, there was one problem – she was three-quarter-scale of an actual northern trawler and simply too small for serious ocean work. Everything about her was smaller than it should have been. The person who designed and built her must have been a midget.

After digging through several layers of rust and the tangle of broken pipes concealing her engine, I was saddened — but not surprised — to discover she was powered by an atomic four-gas engine that would never again rotate. Her machinery resembled a rusty Brillo pad. I would have to replace everything.

But first I had to clean out the fo'c'sle and move in. Paintbrush in hand, I worked to make my new quarters suitable for habitation. By the time I had the forecastle squared away and the engine room cleared out, the afterdeck was piled high with at least a ton of rusty junk. I was afraid of using the dock for temporary storage — it would probably sink under the weight, and it would also block access to the houseboat tied directly behind.

One evening I tossed the entire mess overboard. I was not the first to do so; all the fishing boats at Eychenlob's boat works had been doing the same thing for the past ten years or so. When the tide was low, it was a miracle the boat bottoms cleared the junk pile below.

Obstructing the view from my pipe berth's single porthole was the three-story houseboat, a non-seagoing wreck constructed of uncut sheets of plywood and windows from an old house. The owner of the houseboat was a fast-moving Frenchman, Gene Loba, who was wearing a pair of cutoff shorts so tight he must have used a shoehorn, Vaseline, and a hydraulic jack to force them over his thin frame.

Gene was thrilled to see that the *Restless* had a new owner; one who was young and robust. (I soon understood why he strutted by the *Restless* at every opportunity; his admiration eventually created a problem for me and the woman who became my bride. (More later.)

It took me six weeks to re-power the little trawler with a larger Chrysler Crown engine. Gene was always there to help with a heavy lift, and I helped him pack additional sheets of plywood onto his already overloaded craft. We soon became friends — sort of.

By the time Gene had finished the two upper rooms, the added weight was pressing his craft down into the water by a foot. His sewer pipe, which had originally protruded slightly above the water line, was now submerged. He hadn't used a properly bolted flange while installing the sewer pipe, and the only thing that was keeping the water out was house-caulking, and not much of that.

One evening Gene made the mistake of coming on to one of the tuna fishermen, a strapping thirty-five-year-old with a bad attitude, a drinking problem, and a love for women — not for little Frenchman.

To get back at Gene for making friendly overtures, the tuna fisherman borrowed a huge purse seine skiff with lots of horsepower, and when he uncorked its large inboard engine, the skiff's bow wave was as high as the large skiff itself. The irate fisherman then made several destructive runs past the three-story houseboat. The jarring rocking not only rearranged its interior but also broke the sewer pipe loose, and Gene's home began to sink. Gene was enraged, but he was too busy pumping to do anything about it. I helped by re-caulking the pipe. (This might have been a mistake because Gene became even friendlier.)

Soon after the attack on Gene's home, the *Restless* began to take on water as well. Carl Eychenlob put it on the ways, and I located and easily repaired the leak. I made a sad discovery, however; there was little left of the *Restless's* wooden rudder, and I would have to construct a new one.

I had used up my entire navy leave and could only work weekends. The dry dock fees accrued daily, quickly surpassing my meager wages. I had to hire someone to make the new rudder that same day.

Fat Tommy's abilities as a boat builder were undisputed. He had built his own, fifty-foot fishing boat, the *Sherry*. She was beautiful and well-designed with an aft house. The fish hold and working decks were forward, and he had devised a chute through which he could slide albacore from the rear hatch forward into the hold. Everything he owned was in good order with one exception — his body.

Fat Tommy was short, dark, and very Greek — like Tony — but much younger. Rolls of blubber extended upwards to his ears, camouflaging his once-handsome face. In other words, his head, neck and body were one. He was so fat that, instead of hanging down, his arms stuck almost straight out. And because he had very small feet, he resembled one of Walt Disney's elves. In spite of these obvious handicaps, Tommy was surprisingly speedy and agile.

He appeared to be totally unconcerned about his body, and he loved women. I mean he really loved them! Women would have nothing to do with him, however. The girls in T town even turned their heads when he waddled into their whore houses with a fistful of greenbacks. "Oh no. You too fat. Go 'way."

Tommy constructed a new rudder, painted the bottom, and then launched my trawler — all for no reward. When I returned from my week on the *Nereus*, the *Restless* was once again tied to its dock in front of the houseboat. That night Tommy, Tony, Tommy's boat puller Orlando, Gene and I enjoyed a boat-launching party. Tony prepared the feast, and I happily paid for the grub. We then toasted the handsome little *Restless*. We didn't have clue that we might be, in fact, toasting the devil himself.

Because of my navy duties, the extensive rebuilding of the *Restless* took considerable time. I made money for materials wherever I could. I welded for Carl in his boat works, I did repair work on fishing boats, and I dove for abalone with Lad and Rex. Though I

39

worked hard to finish rebuilding my new toy, the year 1956 had vanished before her slim hull once again felt green water rushing against it.

But when I ran my little jewel through her first sea trials, I became a wiser but sadder student of boat design. Her pilothouse was too low. Though the floorboards were, literally, on top of the engine's spark plugs, I still didn't have room to stand. I could either sit or stand hunched over, like a Viet Nam prisoner in a bamboo cage. After one day at sea, my head was so bruised I looked like I'd been in a street fight. The ghost of the midget boat builder was present, living in her bulges somewhere, enjoying my agony.

I spent as much time as possible at the aft wheel in the rear fish hatch. Here, I was comfortable. However, my forward visibility was blocked by the high bow and pilothouse and, in order to see where I was going on inland waterways, I had to steer from within the wheelhouse. When I arrived back at the dock I looked and sounded older than Tony.

The decks of the *Restless* were smooth and uncluttered. Her rail was but one foot high — just high enough to trip you, head first, into the drink. The only handholds were the two mast stays, one on each side of the pilothouse. Once aft of these, you were on your own. I had to crawl on my hands and knees to survive, in all sea conditions.

It was impossible to get accustomed to her motion. Because of her deep V hull, unlike the round bottoms of most fantails, she had an awkward roll — somewhat like that of a catamaran — a roll with a twist and snap at the end.

Her fore and aft lines were eye-appealing and made her easy to push through the water; however, these same graceful lines caused her to toss violently in a head sea. When the roll and tossing were experienced simultaneously, no seaman on earth could acquire sea legs. Crawling about on all fours while hanging on for your life seemed to be the only answer.

In reverse, she did a ninety-degree turn to port before stopping. My only successful docking technique was to come almost straight in, and very slowly. If I timed it right, reverse kicked her hard to port and the landing was automatic. If the engine died, the landing was followed by a lot of shouting and cursing — the same expressions I used when mooring the *Laura Belle*. And I wasn't the only person doing the shouting and cursing — for the paranoid yacht owners seemed to have no appreciation for such a fine trawler as the *Restless*.

I hated deck engines that clattered and, recalling sea time spent with Rex and Lad, I elected to drive my air compressor off the main engine. Using an auto transmission, I built a power take off and drove it from the front of the Chrysler's flywheel. This put my cast-iron compressor in the fo'c'sle and in the way of my bare feet when I exited my berth. When this occurred, any female companionship I might be enjoying would be driven away by my use of naval adjectives. My lady friends quickly learned an abalone boat was not a yacht, and its owner was not a member of the yacht club.

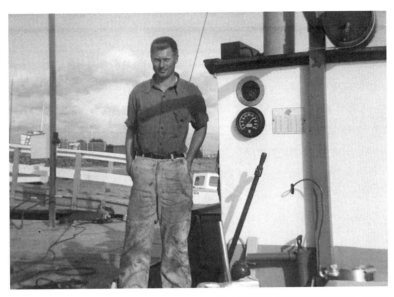

BOB FINISHED WORKING ON THE *RESTLESS* MOTOR, 1957

Tony sympathized with me, my cramped quarters, and my use of language. One evening after drinking too much paisano, he said, "When I was young, the girls thought I was a Greek god. Then they found out I was just a goddamned Greek. I guess you are just a goddamned abalone diver, living in a goddamned abalone boat with a goddamned air compressor." Tony enjoyed swearing even more than me.

The most dangerous challenge to my backyard engineering was the threat to my diving hose from the rotating propeller. I built an adjustable lever to lock the reverse gear in neutral, but because planetary transmissions drag, the prop still rotated slightly. In order to concentrate on my thousand other problems, I convinced myself this was no longer a threat. One day, however, this contraption came back to haunt me; in fact it damn near killed me.

Working hard and saving my pennies, I turned the trawler into an abalone boat. In the process, I learned to master many of her evil ways. Still, by receiving countless blows to the head and bruised knees from crawling, I was constantly reminded that her cursed designer was still on board.

On more than one occasion, I enticed a female along for a ride out to the beautiful kelp beds. Here my fantasy was to enjoy Nature, ala natural. Everytime this situation occurred, my guest would ask to be returned to shore; often right after we had departed. A ride on the *Restless* was simply an ordeal.

41

Every weekend, time and equipment permitting, I would head the trim stem of the *Restless* for the kelp beds off the cavern-filled Ocean Beach cliffs, in search of the elusive abalone. I usually invited one of our navy divers along as a tender; I would teach him to dive for abalone if he would spring for the fish and game license. A good deal for both of us.

Once back on board the navy's *Nereus*, our tales of adventure would have the master divers shaking their heads. Eventually, most of my ideas concerning underwater search and diving equipment would prove more effective and less expensive than those of the navy. But when I was on board the USS *Nereus*, I was considered to be a young kook who was constructing his own diving equipment. A no-no for sure.

Each time we went to sea, I would tie alongside the *Mable* and then visit with Lad and Rex. Lad's brother, Gene Handelman, eventually came west, but he failed to hit it off with Nasty Ed, and the little Frenchman was invited to seek lodging elsewhere. Ed eventually moved into an Ocean Beach apartment and purchased his own boat. Gene then tended Lad and Rex.

The animosity between Ed and Gene ran much deeper than I first realized. One day a dispute arose between them at the boat works, and Ed said something that Gene didn't appreciate. "I'm going to break your leg," Gene responded. The robust man from the Bronx then threw the little Frenchman onto the wooden dock, stepped on his hip, and pulled up hard on his knee. A sharp "CRACK!" could be heard as Ed's femur broke in half. None of us ever learned what had happened between Ed and Gene; neither man ever divulged the basis of their misunderstanding. Some things are better left alone.

A week later we saw Ed out in the kelp beds, pulling his Belle Aqua dry suit up over his cast. It's hell what a man will do when he needs money.

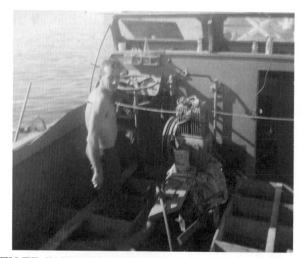

NASTY ED WORKING ON HIS BOAT AT DANA LANDING

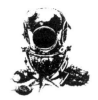

THE CIRCLE INN

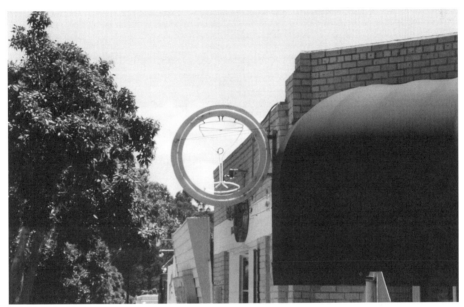

CIRCLE INN

Lad announced he had purchased a live-boat and would be joining Morro Bay's Black Fleet. My discharge date was just around the corner and, once I was a civilian, I planned to drive north, stop at Morro Bay, and toss down a few with Lad and Jerry. Then I would head up to the Bay area and visit my folks. All this was to take place the day I was discharged.

December 1, 1956 – my four-year hitch was over, and I walked down the *Nereus* gangplank for the last time. Some said they were sad to see me leave. My two oldest navy friends, Ed Lawler and Chief Cressie, had long been transferred. My one remaining close friend, Gene Harless, was truly sorry to see me go, but he understood I had plans that did not include Uncle Sam.

Others may have been happy to see me leave. This included Chief Haney who shed few tears. In fact, he had announced that I would be the last second-class diver to actually dive. From then on, second-class divers would be tenders only.

It was great to be a civilian again and, with the world at my fingertips, I was ready for adventure. I had no idea that, within a week, my life would change in a way I could not have imagined.

Early the next morning, after securing the *Restless*, I jumped into my little black

Chevy pickup and headed north towards foggy Morro Bay which is situated about two-thirds the way from San Diego to San Francisco. This little fishing village had two main streets, one traveling east and west and the other, north and south. The old white stucco Circle Inn was on a corner in the middle of town; the equally popular Happy Jack's bar sat kitty-corner, across the street.

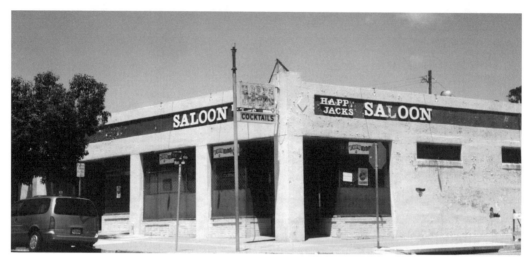

HAPPY JACK'S

A circular shelter — a small roof with a single neon tube around its perimeter — protruded over the always-open front door of the Circle Inn. The young tourist couple who were entering ahead of me stopped dead at the entrance, obviously unable to believe their eyes. Jerry Todd, Ed Wood, and several other divers were perched on the rusty, red naugahyde barstools, having a party. All were naked. Jerry spotted me and the tourists. "Well doggone," he exclaimed. "Come on in, take off your clothes, and have a drink. This here's a nude bar. Bartender, set these folks up."

I sat down next to Ed Wood who, being somewhat less bold than Mr. Todd, had slipped back into his trousers. After I was introduced to all the veteran fisheries divers, I looked around. Several other people were sitting by themselves in corners, and for good reason. One, an older, very well-used gentleman was dressed in dirty khakis. He was introduced as Captain Jet and, for a single drink, he would stand atop a barstool, announce that he was a jet airplane and, with his arms at his sides, dive off. His impact on the wooden floor produced a heavy, slapping "thud/splat!" — a noise resembling the sound of a prizefighter's fist as it connects with the cheek of another prizefighter.

Captain Jet's face bore traumatic evidence — he had obviously been performing this act for years. Then, around midnight every evening, he would curl up in the back door at Happy Jack's and pass out. We raised a toast to Captain Jet, a man who had apparently forgotten his given name. (I was later informed that one night he didn't wake up. He had died, and the janitor had a difficult time mopping around him.)

An abalone diver's tender, Mel Catrel, sat by himself. Mel, a small-framed man in his thirties, bathed but once a year and never changed his clothes until they actually fell off. Sitting near Mel was worse than sitting downwind of a pig farm during the boiling of garbage. Only the less-skilled divers, those who were reduced to scraping the bottom of the barrel, employed Mel. Offering an insight into my early skills, I ended up with this filthy bastard as my regular tender.

Mel's girlfriend was "Three Tit," a noted lady of the evening whose claim to fame was a third udder under her left armpit. Three Tit was a heavily wrinkled member of a local Indian tribe, and she lived in Cambria, a small coastal community north of Morro Bay. Here she was a hustler in a couple of the taverns catering to local low life.

When she was in the mood, she would lift her arm and reveal the hairy vein-lined growth. "Piss on you!" she would cackle before returning to her beer. When she was too drunk to make it to the ladies room, she peed while sitting on the barstool. The bartender didn't seem to mind; he would just mop it up and go back to serving.

We scratched our head, wondering who would pay to have sex with such a beast. Even abalone divers should have had too much class for that.

In the late forties, Barney Clancy had formed Veterans Fisheries with several other divers, most of whom had been in the marines. All boats belonging to Veterans Fisheries were painted black (at one time there were as many as nine) and when they ran together, their presence was demoralizing and the noise, deafening. "Here comes the Black Fleet," the other divers would shout. "We may as well leave."

Ralph Eder, a large diver with a wide grin, was one of the many marine corps vets for whom Barney Clancy had named his Veterans Fisheries. Unlike the other Black Fleet divers, Ralph had poor vision; consequently, he was a slow ab picker. He was, however, steady, reliable, and a joy to work with.

Ralph loved "split-diving" — two divers trading off operating the boat and diving. Though the divers spent only half a day in the water, each earned almost as much as one would earn diving alone. For those of us who were thin and prone to "freezing out" (even when wearing three sets of woolens), this was a good way to go. Once cold, divers like Ralph and me would slow down, becoming most unproductive. I ended up hating the cold Morro Bay waters.

Ralph Eder would sit on a barstool with his head on the bar and snooze. Occasionally he would look up and say, "We don't drink, we don't chew, we don't go with girls who do. Our class won the Bible." Then he would lay his head down for another short nap. (Ralph also told us that he was glad his mother hadn't named him Peter.)

The Circle Inn was probably built right after the war. After fifty years of deferred maintenance, spilled drinks, pee, and vomit, the doors were closed in 1995 for a minor remodel. The name was changed and a new clientele took over. My wife, Claudia, and I stopped by to have a drink a year before the old bar closed and it hadn't changed much since we were there in 1957. Same drunks sitting on the same stool. Happy Jack's was still open, too. It's comforting to know some things never change.

Getting back to my original story. The year is 1956, and I had just been discharged from the navy and was driving up the coast when I stopped at the Circle Inn in Morro Bay. That evening, Jerry invited me out on the town — his idea of a night out was to hit another bar in Cayucos, five miles north. After several beers, I was getting pretty drunk when a very attractive lady walked in — a pleasant surprise because the bar in Cayucos was more sordid than the Circle Inn or Happy Jack's, if that was possible.

The only thing I remember clearly was that she seemed to possess more class than the other women in the establishment. In fact, she appeared to have more class than any of the bar ladies in Morro Bay or Cayucos; a real nice girl with old-fashioned principles; such as not having sex the first hour of a first date.

Drinking too much produces the effect known as "getting drunk." Pulling Jerry's smelly diving wools over my body to stay warm, I retired to the back seat of his Cadillac to sleep it off. I was totally buried in dirty, pungent undergarments when I awoke to voices. The doors at both sides of the front seat opened, and Jerry and the lady with class got in the car. This was followed by much kissing and groaning as things heated up.

"No Jerry," she whispered. "Not here. Let's go to my place around the corner."

"That's fine with me," Mister Todd replied. He then turned to address me. "Is that all right with you, Kirby?"

After putting her bra back on and chewing Jerry out, she walked home and Jerry and I drove to the "ranch house" in Morro Bay.

The ranch house was rented to Barney Clancy by an unsuspecting person who believed abalone divers were normal people. What a rude awakening. The house was ancient and not in good repair but, originally, it had been clean. Now, uncouth divers with their untamed lady friends, wild parties, and dirty diving wools had transformed it, creating chaotic clutter that defied description. The single, very dirty bathroom, was as busy as a ticket office in a New York subway, and the kitchen was piled high with dirty dishes — some which had obviously been sitting there for over a week. The owner could only pray for a fire accompanied by an insurance settlement.

It was free, however, if you were with Veteran's Fisheries. As Jerry's friend who was planning to eventually dive with the outfit, I was welcome to an evening's accommodations.

Such as they were.

Nobody seemed to mind. Actually, the Circle Inn had first priority; in fact, for some of the regulars it appeared to be more of a home than the ranch house.

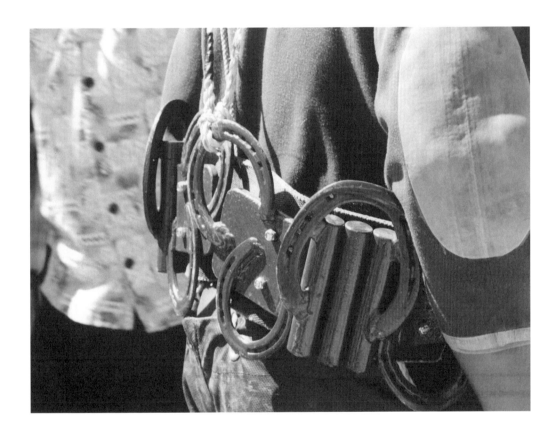

THIS, MY NEW BRIDE, IS THE *RESTLESS*

My trip through Morro Bay also provided me with an opportunity to visit Lad and the Black Fleet. I discovered Lad was very ill and, because he needed to keep bread on the table of his crew, he asked if I could help him and dive his abalone boat for one day. I reluctantly agreed.

His abalone boat — a boat that was very old — was a fantail, the *Pretty Baby*. This craft was well over the hill; only one step better than his uncle's *Sylvia J* in San Diego. Nothing worked well, including the crew. (I grew particularly irritated, later, because Lad dove with this mess everyday and, once I joined the Black Fleet in the spring of 1957, Lad constantly out-picked me.)

Bill Seabright, Lad's operator, was too drunk to stand at the controls, so he sat on a board and hung onto the wheel as if it was his salvation. Lad's tender was not much better — it must have been genetic because he was a first cousin to stinking Mel Catrel.

After I was thirty minutes on the bottom, white slime began running down the inside of the helmet's front port, blocking my view. When I attempted to wipe the goop away with my nose, I succeeded in smearing it all over the glass. As a last resort, forgetting we used mineral oil as our compressor lubricant, I licked it away.

Nature soon called. It was touch and go, getting back on deck and out of the diving dress in time. Adding insult to injury, I ended up with diarrhea for two days and, even more frustrating, the abalone I gathered in my short time on the bottom did little to enhance the salaries of Seabright and the tender; all of this should have been a warning concerning my future as an abalone diver. Unfortunately, I didn't pay attention.

Back on the road, the five-hour drive north stretched into eight, as I was forced to locate rest room facilities along the way — my final payment for spending one day on the *Pretty Babe*. I eventually ended up at my folks' place in Redwood City and, after using their bathroom, I explained my plans. I then called my oldest friend and sailing partner, Tory Imsland. Tory was now a truck driver in Palo Alto, and we agreed to meet at the Hello Club, a dance joint near Atherton. Tory had mustered out of the army the previous year, and we planned to toss down a load of beer while sharing our military experiences and reminiscing about sailing adventures on the San Francisco Bay. At six that evening, the two of us were sitting on barstools near the entrance (and the men's room), engaged in tales of our glorified, daring deeds.

Tory and I had much to discuss, so women were on the back burner. I had noticed a couple of very attractive girls with sailors in the rear of the club but, because they seemed to have escorts, Tory and I didn't pay much attention — a first for me because I loved women. (A divers curse?)

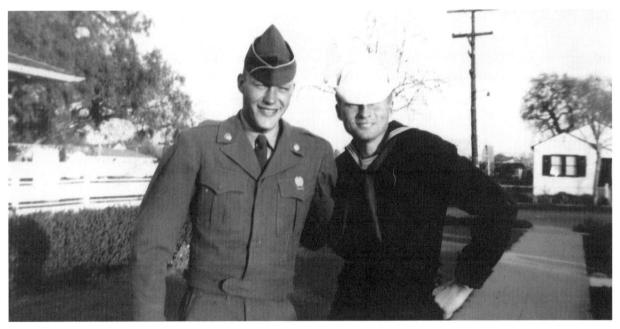

TORY AND BOB, 1954

Unknown to us, the sailors — after outgrowing their welcome — had left the scene, and now the girls were heading toward the front entrance. As they passed, Tory recognized one — a girl he had met the previous evening at an army buddy's wedding, and the girls accepted the invitation to join us in a brew and conversation.

The girl Tory had recognized, the more attractive of the two, sat next to me and introduced herself as Claudia. She was (still is!) a knockout — blue-eyed, tall and thin with a gorgeous figure. That moment, and all moments to follow, I completely forgot about Tory. Fifteen minutes after our initial meeting, I asked her to marry me and she accepted.

Tory, in total shock, was asked to take Claudia's friend home, and Claudia and I — in her little red MG roadster — drove back to Redwood City where I introduced her to my parents. While there, we had hot tea and finalized our plans. I would pick her up at her apartment at seven the next evening, and we would drive to Half Moon Bay to see her folks. We would then leave for San Diego where we would drop off her belongings on the *Restless* before heading to Yuma to get married.

Once back in San Diego, our next chapter would be a lifetime adventure with the ocean, and I would teach her the ways of the sea. Unfortunately, I would soon learn that she was a confirmed landlubber, with farm dirt under her fingernails.

My future bride had many problems to take care of before our seven o'clock appointment. She had to arrange for a leave of absence from her job, terminate her apartment rental, pack her belongings, attend to a long list of errands, and keep her dental appointment for a root canal.

When I pulled up in front of her apartment the following evening, she was hardly the carefree person I had met the previous evening. Instead, she was now running on pure adrenaline. Then, when her ex-boyfriend spotted us loading my pickup, he wanted to know what was up. She shined him on with some silly excuse, and we made our departure.

Claudia's dad, the principal at Half Moon Bay High, was very concerned. "You're an abalone diver?" he asked. When I told him I planned to take his beautiful daughter out on the ocean in a boat I had rebuilt himself, he grew even more upset.

Her parents wanted to know how long we had known one another. Claudia responded with a merciful white lie. "Oh," she hesitated, "about two months."

We departed Half Moon Bay around nine that evening to dutiful farewell waves, then drove perhaps one hundred miles south to King City on Highway 101, emotionally bushed. I'm sure the man at the motel desk didn't believe us when we told him we were married and too weary for sleep, or anything else.

We were strangers when we awakened the next morning, but by the end of the day we were referring to one another by silly names. The foolish names were necessary because I had forgotten Claudia's given name. (When she was in the rest room, I went through her wallet in order to recall it.)

At Eychenlob's in San Diego, I took Claudia by the hand, led her down the twisted and sinking docks, and introduced her to our beautiful little trawler. The *Restless* was just as I had left her, in shipshape condition. We stowed her possessions in the fo'c'sle, next to the air compressor. I failed to inform her that there was no way to lock the boat, but who would enter it anyway? Nothing aboard was of any actual value, just my diving gear and her belongings. When I introduced her to Tony, he assured her he would keep an eye on things. I didn't tell her that he drank gobs of wine every evening.

I had observed Gene Loba, watching us from his third-story window as we unloaded Claudia's things. He had avoided us when we passed in the parking lot, an indication that he disapproved of my future mate.

In Yuma, the gentleman in the reversed collar informed us that if we wanted to get married, we had to hurry because he had another appointment. Still wearing our wrinkled and sweaty traveling clothes, Claudia and I said our vows, found a restaurant, located a motel, and − for the first time in three days − we relaxed.

What a body...

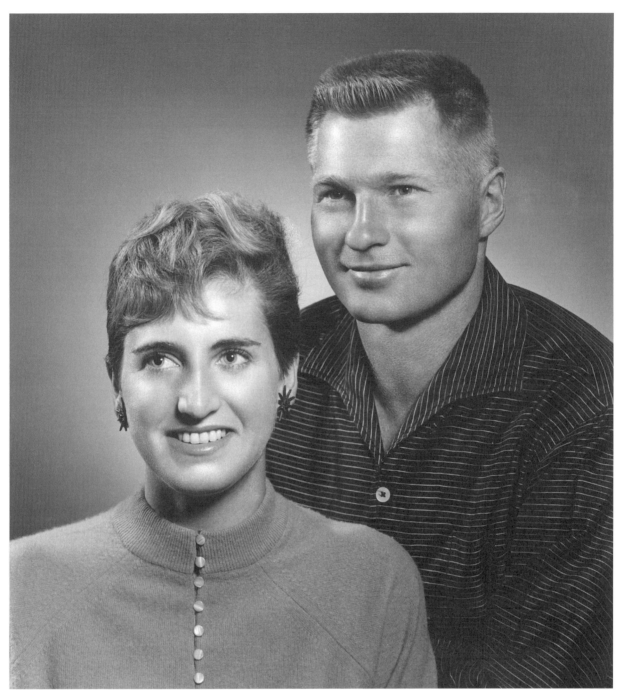

CLAUDIA AND BOB, 1956

Our return to the *Restless* was not as joyful as we had hoped for, after removing the fo'c'sle floorboards, someone had shoved my bride's clothing into the oily bilge water. She wanted to cry but maintained her composure and, after loading her clothing into the truck, we headed for a laundromat.

The following day I dropped our extension cord, the cord feeding power from the shore, into the water. Gene's high-fi, a large black box filled with radio tubes, was on the same circuit, and the delicate tones of classical music were instantly replaced by loud and ugly garbles. Gene burst out of his houseboat and ran down the dock until he came to the cord, now boiling in the salt water. After jerking it out, he beat it to death by pounding it on the wooden planks. When I began to chuckle, Claudia gained her first insight into my warped sense of humor. She has been a little leery ever since.

Mrs. Olsen, in her twilight years, rented us an apartment in Ocean Beach for eighty dollars a month and, because we moved in on a Saturday, the gas wouldn't be turned on until Monday. Undaunted, Claudia returned from the market with an armload of salad ingredients. I had no idea I had married a cook. The salad was great, and we topped it off in the sack. Things don't get much better than that.

The next day I began introducing her to my friends. Nasty Ed lived only a block away, so he was first. When he opened his door we caught sight of the largest stack of dirty laundry Claudia had ever seen. His clothing reeked of abalone juice and engine oil and, since we had washing facilities in our new apartment, I volunteered Claudia as an angel of mercy. (She later told me she counted seventy-four shirts and twenty-seven pairs of Levi's – good thing Ed never wore underwear or socks.) When washed and folded, Ed's laundry filled the bed of the pick-up.

The following morning, a perplexed Mrs. Olsen approached. "Claudia," she asked, "are you taking in laundry?" Claudia explained that she had done the washing for free and that it was my idea. Then she called me a stupid jerk.

How quickly her explicit vocabulary had expanded since we first arrived at the fish docks.

THIS IS AN ABALONE

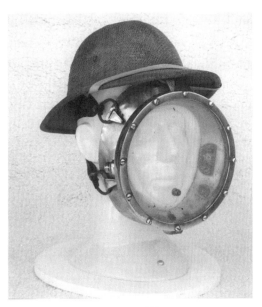

#1 MASK

I knew I couldn't take Claudia out into the ocean completely unprepared and, at first, I attempted to talk her into becoming a diver. I wanted her to at least try it; then she would appreciate what it feels like to walk on the ocean floor, surrounded by the cool, beautiful liquid environment. She would begin by diving in ten feet of water at the boat works where I could tend her from the deck of the *Restless*. I just knew she would love it.

After persuading her to wear her bikini (considered to be very revealing in the late 50s), I enticed her to don my stainless steel mask, then make her way down the diving ladder. Looking back, I'm not sure what I was thinking of or trying to accomplish. I guess I just wanted to show off her great body. If I really wanted her to become a diver, why did I pick this particular spot for her first lesson?

Everyone was watching. Tony was sitting on the fish hatch of the *Antone*; Fat Tommy was on the high bow of the *Sherry* where he could watch Claudia's every motion and wiggle; all the customers at the restaurant above the boat works were on the back deck. I could have sold tickets.

When Claudia's feet were placed on the ladder, all cheered. As soon as her breasts were submerged, they were taking bets. And when she went under and didn't burst to the surface, some of the losers had to pay off.

53

Once she was under she gripped the ladder's rung tight enough to remove the paint, and I reached down to pry her hands off so she could descend deeper. She gripped the next rung even harder and, because this was too deep for me to reach, I took off my shoes, climbed down the ladder and, encouraging her to let go, I stood on her hands.

Instead, she burst to the surface above me and, mask in hand and dripping, she let me have it. It appeared to me that Claudia was turning out to have very thin skin. Perhaps she really didn't want to be a diver. (Or have her fingers mashed.)

The crowd at the restaurant was still laughing as they returned to their tables, and I overheard one customer say, "Diving instructor, my butt. That red-headed newlywed will be lucky to get any by the end of this month!"

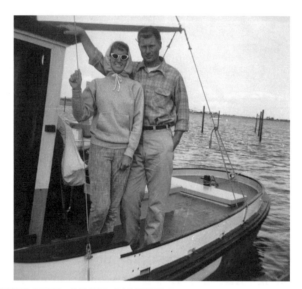

THE TWO OF US ON THE *RESTLESS*, MAY 1957

After two more days of maintenance, the three of us − Claudia, our abalone boat, and me − were ready for the magical experience the ocean had to offer. The morning was calm, and our trawler rolled in its inimitable, devil-inspired style off the Point Loma cliffs as the sun's early warming rays burned off the remaining fog.

I located an area containing plenty of kelp with an indication of rocks at the bottom. I sounded the depth − sixty feet − which was just right. I dropped anchor, set back on it, took the engine out of gear, and pulled on my new wetsuit. Claudia sat on the fish hatch, awaiting my command.

As I got on the ladder, I realized I had not set the safety pin into the lever which prevented the reverse gear from engaging the propeller. If I didn't take care of this I could be dragged across the bottom like a fishing weight, so I asked Claudia to set it. "Okay hon,"

54

she said, smiling as she came out of the wheelhouse. "The pin's in."

It occurred to me that she had taken quite a long time to set the pin, but she was new at this. Then I had her secure my mask and the rubber "spider" holding it to my head. Forgetting to make sure my hose was snapped into my belt, I bailed into the water with a huge splash from high on the ladder, a demonstration designed to assure Claudia she had not married a wimp.

The sea floor quickly rose up to meet me. What visibility! I could see forever, and the bottom was magnificent. Rocks were everywhere, and the one right in front of me held at least a dozen abalone. We would be raking them in today!

Suddenly, my mask was ripped from my face in an explosive blast of bubbles and seawater. Instinctively, I grabbed for it, replaced it, and re-fastened the spider. Next, I snapped my hose into my belt as I should have done in the first place. Finally, I looked up. My hose was running at a shallow angle, not up as it should have been running. I realized the *Restless* was underway; instead of setting the lock pin into the lever, Claudia had set the adjustment handle which resembled the lock pin. This then engaged the engine into forward gear.

My next moves would prove to be a severe test of my faith and my endurance. I was off and running, a scared animal being pursued for slaughter, over the rock-covered bottom. I had to run or be dragged through the sharp and spiny sea life – beautiful bottom my butt.

I lost my abalone bag between a couple of rocks, but I certainly didn't care. I was worried for my life, not a bag of twine and hose. Outfitted with heavy weights and shoes instead of swim fins, I was rigged for walking, but I questioned my ability to swim any distance. In a struggle to reach the surface, I began climbing my hose, hand over hand. All three-hundred feet of my hose was over the side; thank God I had tied it off to a deck cleat to relieve the strain or it would have already parted company with its air fitting, leaving me and my hose far behind. My bride would then be steaming off into the fog in an abalone boat divorced from its skipper.

I considered bailing out of my weights and swimming toward the surface while attempting to ignore my walking shoes, but then I would come up somewhere far behind the boat. The boat and Claudia would continue to power on while I drowned in an attempt to catch them. Bailing out was, obviously, a very poor option.

I thanked God for the machete we divers carry to cut the pea kelp. Doubling as an abalone bar and measuring tool, I could now use it to slash at the endless green forest that stood between me, sunshine, and air.

I climbed using both hands, heavy-duty chin-ups, one after another; pull, hold, reach higher, pull again, rest, repeat. Hanging on with my left hand, I would hack at the forest of kelp with the other. I imagine I harvested an acre of the slimy stuff but, as I chopped, it would float back and collect in the lengthening bight of my air hose. The mass could be compared to a giant sea anchor, doing its best to pull me back and keep me from moving up towards the surface.

The game seemed to go on forever — pull, hold, slash, pull again. As spots formed in front of my eyes, I prayed to my Maker. (It flashed on me — I was sure the night spent in Tijuana with the twin sisters, two years earlier, wiped out any Brownie points I might have accumulated.) As the spots before my eyes grew brighter, I called upon my ancestors, all the time pulling and slashing in a nightmarish trance.

Then, there it was! The bottom rung of my ladder! With a desperate and possibly last burst of energy, I reached for it, hung on, and when the spots had disappeared, I looked around. The propeller of the trawler was turning at a nice pace, pushing us along at about two knots. Still anchored, we had cut a five-hundred-foot circle through the kelp. It was as if I had harvested a circular alfalfa farm in the California desert, all by myself.

But my struggle wasn't over. I still had to climb up that ladder, and this required two more pull-ups before I could get my knees on the bottom rung. Until my chin was actually on the rail, I wasn't sure I would survive.

My bride removed my spider and mask. She stood there in the sun, wearing her small swimsuit and smiling like an angel. "Is there anything wrong, Hon?"

As the day progressed, the tension remained. Claudia was now expressing reservations about a life at sea. Measuring the abalone and heaving a full bag aboard was difficult, and she constantly fretted about the little details — air pressure and our anchor. The near-disaster certainly hadn't helped.

By the end of the day it was obvious she needed a little moral support and I decided to ask Knox to tend for a couple of days. As an expert, perhaps he could help defuse her building anxiety.

"I don't like the naked parties at Knox's place," Claudia had informed me earlier. "We're not swingers." However, she did like the man who hosted these wild events. She appreciated his laid-back personality and sense of humor. And she got to know him even better the following day. As the fog burned off the next morning, the *Restless* held three occupants instead of two and life was looking good. Or so it seemed at the time.

We anchored in the same area, and Claudia sat on the fish hatch and watched Knox help me into my gear. This time I checked everything carefully. Our air pressure was up and the reversing handle had been properly secured — the propeller shaft was not turning. The old Chrysler was counting out its slow and even cadence without missing a beat. The ocean was flat, and the water appeared to have as much visibility as it had the previous day. I would gather a good harvest and Knox would do the same. Things seemed to be going our way and, if they stayed that way, our trawler would be paid off in a week.

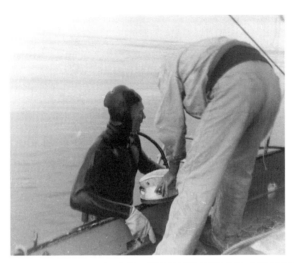

KNOX HARRIS TENDING BOB IN SAN DIEGO, JANUARY 1957

I dropped in and the bottom again rose up to greet me, as beautiful as it had been a day earlier. Streaks of light created by shafts between the flowing kelp foliage extended downward, and with each movement of the soft swell the colors at the bottom changed. With each surge, the canopy of vegetation swayed. I felt as if I was moving in slow motion, and the problems of the world above seemed terribly insignificant. Sport diving was a very new sport in the late 1950s, and I was observing a wonderful world few people had ever seen. I knew I was one of the privileged few.

Back on deck, Knox was sunbathing on top of the small wheelhouse while Claudia attempted to relax on the fish hatch, knowing that Knox was ready and able to overcome any obstacle that might arise.

The gods were being good, and my bag was almost completely filled with deep reds; the reds would bring far more money than the pinks because they were much larger and had more meat. It was going to be a great day.

Suddenly, my hose became taut as if, once again, I was being pulled off the bottom. I was not just going up, I was being rapidly pulled in. I was surrounded by kelp which I couldn't cut fast enough. I soon lost my last abalone bag, and it was full.

I neared the bottom of the *Restless*; things looked normal. The propeller was motionless and I could see the anchor line which meant we were still well-anchored. What could be wrong? Why would they pull me up so fast? I grew angry. What was the matter with my crew? Had Knox lost his mind? I had lost a large bag filled with abalone and would probably never see it again. What was going on?

57

Claudia was yelling at me as she removed my mask. "Down-there-in-the-fo'c'sle,-down-there!!!" She was talking so fast her words didn't make any sense.

"Dammit," I exclaimed, "why the hell did you pull me up so fast? I lost my last bag."

"Because of the mess in the fo'c'sle," she answered.

"What mess?"

"Over here! Down there! Look! I know something is wrong, I just know it!" She appeared panic-stricken, and Knox was very upset as well.

"Good grief, Kirby, what a mess. I have no idea what happened."

I peered down the scuttle and into the dark fo'c'sle housing the compressor. It resembled a lumberyard that had been hit by a tornado. My pipe berth was all twisted up, the wooden seats were torn apart, and my air compressor — laying on its side — was missing its flywheel.

Oh no...the flywheel broke free and in its erratic flight damn near sank the Restless before dying in the bottom of the fo'c'sle.

There the flywheel lay, partially hidden under the scattered woodpile. If it had gone through the bottom planks of our little boat, we would have been forced to swim ashore. This had been a very close call.

After a thorough inspection, we discovered the compressor's crankshaft had, at one time, been broken, then welded. The weld had failed, and the flywheel had performed as it was designed to perform; it had continued to rotate until it ran out of energy. The fo'c'sle had to be rebuilt and the crankshaft replaced before we could do any more diving. Any hope of paying off the little boat by the end of year had now — like the boat itself almost — been dashed against the rocks.

The best we could hope for was to repair it and get in one week of diving before the season ended. Crap happens, and it often comes in a rusty fifty-gallon drum labeled, "Lots of Crap."

Cashing in her one remaining savings bond, Claudia paid for a new crankshaft and lumber to rebuild the fo'c'sle, and in a week we were once again ready for the sea. We were also on our own, for Knox had to return to his lifeguarding duties.

We spent one hard week, doing our best to make money. The previously superb bottom visibility was now ruined by a rolling, northwesterly swell, and each day was worse than the day before. We were getting abalone, but not enough. We needed one more big haul — one load to help us through the two-month off-season that was just days away.

The answer was simple. We would run a load of shorts, filling our hold if we could. To avoid getting caught, we would unload at the boat works and truck our abalone to Eli's when it was dark.

Abalone need clean cool water, a surge, and adequate feed to prosper. When there is a shortage of food, the abalone are stunted, creating a short bed. This results in a large population of underfed abalone never reaching legal size. One such short bed was discovered out to sea off the very tip of Point Loma where there was very little kelp. The abalone here were mainly shorts, and there were lots of them.

On the last morning of the season — our last chance to make our final stake — the abalone gods were smiling once again. There was just enough fog to hide us from the view of the fish cop — the same guy who had caught Jerry earlier. I knew he would love to put us in the slammer, for he would surely remember me.

In four hours we had quite a load. I thinned the bed in a random pattern to allow the remaining mollusks to grow. We piled our few legal abalone on the deck; then we shucked the rest, placed them in gunny sacks, and stored them in the fish hold. Under cover of darkness, we used a wheelbarrow to transport our booty to the black Chevy pickup. We had concealed everything with canvas including smelly fishnets and an assortment of items from the boat works.

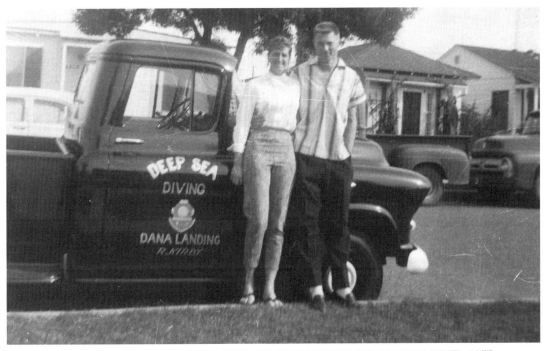

BOB AND CLAUDIA IN FRONT OF OCEAN BEACH APARTMENT, 1957

As we drove into Eli's, we spotted the damned fish cop talking to the fish processor. "Quick, Claudia," I said, "move over against me as close as possible. Make like we're lovers on a tour." I actually stopped in front of the two men to point out objects of interest. The uniformed cop missed us, but I was covered with sweat for the next couple of hours.

We unloaded later, then beat it out of there.

The money I received for the undersized meat was hardly worth the effort. I spent the next six weeks in a shipyard, welding, until we could afford to take up diving again. What a great occupation.

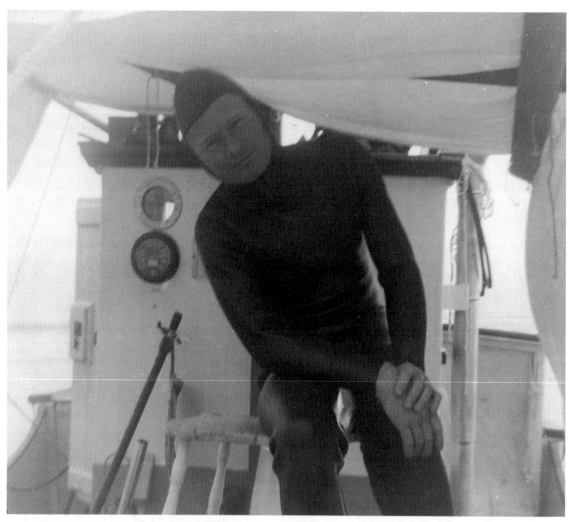

"MAN FROM MARS" PREPARING TO INVADE POOR LITTLE ABS IN SAN DIEGO

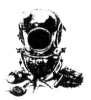

HEY WHITE MAN, HOW COME YOU'RE SO MEAN?

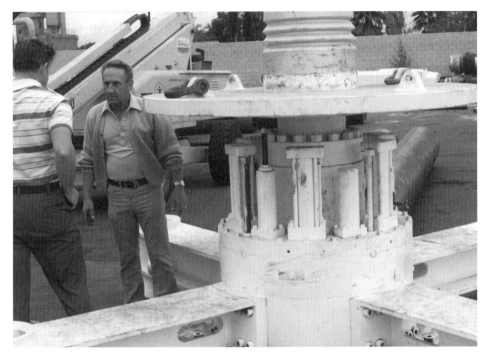

WHITEY, 1980

Jerry drove to San Diego to visit us before partying in Ocean Beach, and he offered me the use of the *Sea Deuce* for the 1957 season in Morro Bay. He had promised Whitey Stefens the boat but Whitey hadn't shown up — he had probably decided to continue lobster fishing in San Pedro. Jerry needed someone he could trust and his younger brother, D.C. Todd, wanted to split-dive with me, a situation made in heaven. Jerry figured D.C. and I would be glad to dive the *Sea Deuce*, and he was correct. All we had to do was show up a month before the season began, clean up the boat, put new diving gear aboard, and go for it. A supposed piece of cake that evolved into one month of back-breaking, dirty work.

My immediate problem was the *Restless*. What would I do about my own boat? I came up with the bright idea of leasing it to Rex who could find another diver and make a buck for us while we were in Morro Bay. It didn't occur to me that Rex, who was much taller than me, would end up hating the tiny trawler more than I did. (I later discovered hack marks in the overhead beams where Rex had vented his anger with his abalone bar. Then, after beating the hell out of the beams, he took the remainder of his foul mood out on the rest of the boat. And I didn't blame him.)

Claudia and I rented a lovely, rustic apartment on a pine-covered hill overlooking the town of Morro Bay. We found the *Sea Deuce* on the ways at the Morro Bay Boat Works, surrounded by many of the other boats belonging to the Black Feet.

At first glance, aside from needing paint, she appeared to be in good condition. After further inspection, however, we discovered a host of small repairs that needed to be taken care of before she would be ready for another year at sea. For instance, her steering cables were frayed and needed to be replaced. She also needed a good cleaning, inside and out. We would be lucky to finish these jobs in the month before opening day and still have time for sea trials.

I had met D.C. Todd earlier. He was a splendid young man — eager and intelligent — and we soon had the *Sea Deuce* back in the water. As a member of Clancy's Black Fleet, she was now sporting a coat of fresh black paint.

That was a particularly memorable month in my life. In order to have the boats and gear ready by March 15, the first day of the season, we were all very busy. I loved working on the boats, and the small boat works was a beehive of activity. The other Black Fleet divers and crew members were hard at it — painting, replacing gear, and maintaining their vessels. Harold Elmore and Frank Brebe had their own processing plant, and the men working for them were just as busy.

Laddie and his operator, Bill Seabright, were also consumed, but because Bill remained steadfastly drunk, I don't know how Laddie managed to get his boat ready in time. Had it not been for George Rebuck's assistance, outfitting the *Pretty Babe* with diving gear, I'm sure Lad would not have made it.

One of the more unusual crafts in the yard was a very old, nineteen-foot dory that looked as if it was straight off the decks of a New England sailing schooner. I asked the yard foreman where the boat came from, and the man in dirty coveralls laughed. "Who knows?" he replied. "Some jerk going by the name 'Captain Jim Penn' had her shipped from the east coast. He wants to be an abalone diver; said he read about it in a magazine he found in the Galt, Kansas, library." When he told me this, I began laughing to myself, never suspecting Captain Jim Penn would be entering my life.

I grew to know the Black Fleet divers and their crews — great men — many of whom were veterans of WWII. Some, like Jerry and me, had learned to dive in the navy. Others were former marines; many of them had attended the Sparling School of Diving and Underwater Welding in Wilmington, California, after they were mustered out of the service.

These ex-GIs were the core of Veteran's Fisheries Black Fleet. They would do anything to assist the other divers and I welcomed their support. Many remain friends today, while others have moved on to the big abalone bed in the sky.

I installed the Japanese helmet that I had converted aboard the *Nereus*, and we were ready for sea trials. I was surprised how quickly D.C. learned to operate our vessel. He was good, very good, and so was I. The *Sea Deuce* could turn on a dime. She was a joy to operate.

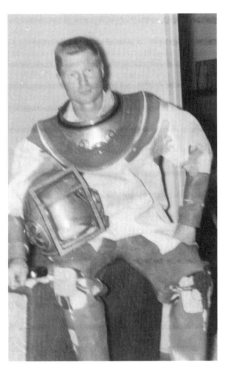

BOB WITH THE JAPANESE HELMET, JANUARY, 1957

This generation of boats was far more versatile than the older Monterey-built Siino boats used by the Japanese; boats that had almost no accommodations. However, they operated well because the small aft-mounted pilot house weathervaned the boat's bow into the oncoming wind. A single sculling oar in the stern powered its ancestor. Then, in the twenties, single-cylinder engines were installed. Engines that were more powerful soon followed and, in the thirties and forties, the small aft living quarters appeared. There was a downside to these, for the forward decks were now exposed to the waves and head seas.

Our design, with the house and flying bridge forward, worked against us, weathervaning us away from the wind and oncoming swells. However, with our powerful engines and a little practice, we were able to overcome this problem.

Our boats offered the best of all worlds. They were faster, had very good accommodations, and the aft deck work area was dry. They could also carry large loads, eliminating the need for a pick-up boat.

It would be a good year. I would not freeze as I did in San Diego because we would now be in dry, heavy gear. My partner was smart and reliable, and we could learn to live with our less-than-clean tender, Melvin C. Catrel, whom we had hired straight from the Circle Inn.

Don Gallagher, who dove the *Cathy*, was usually high boat; Ed Wood on the *Lorraine W* was second. Most of the other boats were also ahead of us, but just barely. Our loads were fairly decent — perhaps fifteen dozen to Don and Ed's twenty. D.C. and I had little to complain about. We were making a buck and enjoying the last of the sunny, spring conditions in Morro Bay.

Winter's end always brings clear weather, broken only occasionally by a brief storm. Summer is different. No storms, just the "June Gloom," a consistent fog which is usually accompanied by a stiff breeze with its freezing chop — as miserable as is possible.

Our daily schedule was simple. In order to be at the beds in time, I got up at five, had breakfast, then headed down to the *Sea Deuce*. D.C. was always there when I arrived, and we left the dock at seven. In the evening we would head home at four, arrive at five, and, by the time we had unloaded, washed down and fueled, it was six-thirty. At the time this did not seem to be a particularly long day. If our pace was broken every couple of weeks, it was because of nature's high seas, not because our will to work had been weakened.

Claudia found employment at Bob's Sea Foods where she served fish and chips. Our meager savings had been exhausted during the overhaul time and, when I occasionally helped at the restaurant, we could eat for nothing. I would peel spuds for the French fries, filling in for their regular peeler, Mel Catrel, who was often drunk. (No one understood why the seldom-bathed Mr. Catrel always had clean hands until we discovered he had been peeling potatoes the night before.)

Except for a few days of large swells, we kept up the *Sea Deuce* pace of diving for two months. Our bank account began to flourish, a first for Claudia and me. Then one evening when we arrived at Clancy's dock, we were met by a short, blonde-haired man with a badly damaged nose. He wasn't smiling.

He watched while we unloaded and cleaned the *Sea Deuce*. "Are you Bob Kirby?" he shouted when we were finished.

"Yeah," I answered. "I'm Kirby."

"And is the other man D.C. Todd?"

"Yes, dammit. He is."

"Good. Be here at five and be fueled up."

D.C. stopped what he was doing and looked at me. "Is that jerk Whitey Stefens? If so, we'll have to fire Mel."

The following morning, the three of us were on the *Sea Deuce* at five as Whitey had commanded. (Claudia wasn't too happy about making my breakfast and lunch at four in the morning.)

Not a word passed between the three of us as we headed the *Sea Deuce* out the Morro Bay channel, and things stayed that way all day. We were not even sure if this man <u>was</u> Whitey — he never introduced himself. Then, as I dressed him in, I asked if we were going to be able to dive as well. "Sure," he said. "When I'm tired."

He never tired, however. A little dynamo, he would get on the bottom while it was still so dark he could barely see and, with the exception of surfacing for a brief lunch, he would not come up until it was so late he couldn't distinguish a rock from an abalone. If the winter days hadn't been so short, we probably would have remained in the kelp until our fuel ran out.

There was a bright side. We always came in with a good load, and we were never lower than the other top boats. Though our cut wasn't bad, D.C. and I did not make as much money has we had when we were diving. I also missed my wife and regretted spending so much time with Whitey Stefens, our seldom-content diver. He was the most intense man I've ever known; no one could beat him. He rarely spoke and occasionally he acted with his fists. I wondered how he and his former partner, Jimmy Pirog, managed not to kill one another.

Unlike Jimmy, however, Whitey took good care of his boat, machinery, and diving gear. He liked things to be clean, well thought-out, and correctly done. This was one characteristic Whitey and I shared, and we eventually became somewhat friendly. On the other hand, I may be overstating our relationship a tad.

A master in heavy gear, Whitey taught us many new tricks. For instance, he rolled up a small rag and put it on the hat's view port shelf; then he placed his nose on the rag so as to blow and clear his ears. He explained how he arrested a free descent by bending over and then, by turning up his air for an instant, he could trap a large pocket of air in the back of his dress. To descend, he straightened up and bumped his helmet's internal exhaust valve. Instead of climbing a line or hose, Whitey ascended the same way. As I said before, after a couple of weeks we almost grew to like him.

As the weeks passed, D.C. and I never got wet. We did, however, gain much experience tending and operating. One thing we learned was the value of hard work. Both of us enjoyed goofing off, so our work habits had been somewhat frayed. Whitey forced us both to clean up our act.

(Whitey mellowed over the years, and I grew a lot wiser. We became the best of friends, see one another regularly, and a few years ago when he was rebuilding a boat, I worked for him as a welder.)

65

As I prepared steaks that evening, I told everyone within earshot (including Whitey) about the work D.C. and I had done on the *Sea Deuce* and, and how this little jerk had shown up to take over.

"For two cents," I said, "I'd wipe myself with his steak."

Whitey took one bite. "Tastes like you already did."

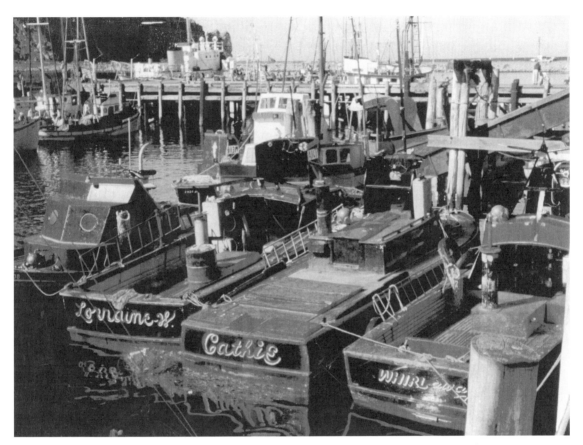

Steve Rebuck

BLACK FLEET, MORRO BAY

Desperate to get back in the water, I decided to quit the *Sea Deuce* and acquire my own boat. Looking back, this was a stupid move because Whitey only stayed another month before heading home to fish lobsters again, and D.C. found another guy to split-dive with and rehired Mel. For a reason I will never know, my diving gear remained on the *Sea Deuce*, and I never saw it again.

To make matters even worse, the boat I ended up buying — with money I had borrowed from Barney — turned out to be a piece of junk. (Forty-five years later, my bride still brings this up. I can't blame her, for she didn't like the idea of my borrowing from Barney in the first place and told me so in rather vivid terms.)

But first I had considered rebuilding the *Restless*. "We can replace her midget pilot house with an open, flying bridge. She's slow, but seaworthy."

I could tell Claudia wasn't convinced; for that matter, neither was I. We had to do something with the little trawler, however. We had just received a note from Rex. He had moved back to his hometown to build houses, and the *Restless* was once again tied up at Eychenlob's boat works.

We found her in need of much cosmetic repair, for Rex had once again relieved his rage with an abalone bar. It took a week of filling, sanding, and painting to get her back as nice as the day Rex had received her. I gave up my foolish plan to rebuild the *Restless*, and I sold her the following day.

Her new owner was even taller than Rex. I was positive he would quickly come to hate the fantail, and the *Restless* would hate him with equal vengeance. I later learned he removed the engine in order to make headroom in the wheelhouse and relocated the engine in the fish hold. Now useless for commercial fishing, the *Restless* spent her final days as a pleasure craft.

Wooden boats are not merely planks and nails. Once launched, they assume a soul and become living things with temperaments and personalities, good and bad. Clancy's black boats were all user-friendly. They operated well and didn't display strange tendencies such as the *Restless*'s habit of swapping ends when in reverse. Clancy's boats didn't break down every other day. Instead, they were reliable, nice to live on when aboard, and they didn't sink once a week. These were the qualities we were looking for when we decided to buy another boat, but the pickings were slim. In Morro Bay, only one boat fitting our requirements was available, the *Rosy*, and then my criteria would be stretched to the limits.

The *Rosy* was built by the Montgomery brothers in the forties and was actually a pointed barge. Her duties included being towed to Lion Rock to be loaded with sea gull guano which was a valued fertilizer. Designed for ease in towing, she had pleasant lines and was well built, a necessity because the *Rosy* frequently ended up on the rocks. When this took place, she would be towed into the harbor, beached at high tide, rolled on her side, and repaired before the next incoming tide.

Morro Bay is not known for having tropical weather. The *Rosy's* cold evening repairs − hasty and crude − were assisted by a warming solution known as bourbon. Her planks had no ribs supporting their ends − they merely floated, secured by oakum caulking and sheet lead patches. Who cared? She was just a barge.

When the guano supply ran out, the *Rosy* was given a new life and became an abalone boat. Using the same exacting standards, the team who had been repairing her were involved in her conversion. Their primary assisting fluid remained bourbon − lots of it − and they used concrete − even more of this − to stabilize the floating planks.

Over the years, many divers had graced the *Rosy's* leaking decks, including George Veramonte who put himself through college, diving from the relic. George had expended little effort on maintenance, especially during his last year on board, and though the old boat was forlorn, she was available — diving gear and all — for $2000 as is, where is. With my check from Barney Clancy in hand, I'm sure George laughed all the way to the bank. Barney's words still ring in my ears: "Okay, but the boat is yours. YOU fix the son of a bitch and YOU pay for it." Barney was no fool.

When I took the *Rosy* out for a spin, I was surprised at the speed the converted Buick-eight gave her. Her pointed bow, low profile, and amidships plywood house resisted any tendency to be blown off by the wind, and she was steady as a rock. On the other hand, she had the turning radius of a freight train.

I soon discovered why she was so steady — the concrete in her bilges was responsible for the unusual engine room substructure. The Montgomery brothers had poured a large amount of concrete here in order to settle her flopping plank ends and prevent them from leaking. Thank God she had a powered Jabsco bilge pump that was able to throw water twenty feet, a pump that she constantly needed in order to remain afloat.

On each side of her engine was a shallow bathtub formed of the rock-like substance. When water leaked in from her decks, and it always did, I had to mop it up or I would get wet feet when I worked on the engine or went forward. This was a non-ending nuisance.

Her diving gear consisted of a rather decent Desco sponge hat with a very small face port. The old helmet had phones that barely worked, and I would have to replace them both as soon as possible. The diving shoes were rusty, steel parts that had been welded together. The compressor was a well-used Quincy that produced sixteen cubic feet per minute. (This was a model everyone used.) The compressor was driven off the front of the Buick and was mounted on a rusty plate that had seen better days — perhaps twenty years worth.

I would have loved to strip away her dowdy house and build a new one, but I needed the money so diving before the repairs had been made was a necessity. Everything else would have to wait until we were blessed with rough seas and high swells and couldn't access the abalone grounds. For the time being, the seas were flat and I would have to use the *Rosy* as she was.

Crew members not already employed were hardly worth hiring. I located Mel, long ago fired by D.C., sitting on his usual bar stool at the Circle Inn. I found "Laughing Bob" Long at home; Bob was a wonderful operator but his continual laughter drove people nuts. What the hell...dirty Mel who stunk, Laughing Bob who could make a preacher lay down his Bible, me wearing a helmet with a small view port and weak phones — all of us packed together in a leaking guano barge powered by a rusty, aging car engine whose days were numbered. I was really learning to love this business.

A swell came up overnight, and the next morning my boat struggled to clear the rock jetty. Bob knew the ropes — count three large sets, then duck out and around the end of the rock wall on the chance the fourth swell would be low.

As we approached the jetty, nature called. I lowered our half-filled deck bucket on a rope and into the center of the starboard concrete bathtub which placed me next to the clattering Buick engine. Then I climbed down the ladder, dropped my pants, and sat on the bucket with my feet tangled in the deck rope in front. I was preparing to pull up my trousers and dump the bucket's contents overboard when Bob rounded the rocks, and an unexpectedly large swell lifted our bow at a very steep angle. I lost my balance, stepped on the rope, and the contents of the bucket ended up inside my Levi's and down around my feet.

After climbing out of my soggy soiled clothing and into my wools, I had to mop up the mess sloshing around in the bottom of the tub.

Bob was laughing all the time — his infernal laugh — even while I was chewing him out for not keeping my tender downwind during the dressing-in procedure. And if I thought Mel smelled bad? He certainly had nothing on me that day.

We saw low production and little profit that week because the *Rosy* couldn't turn tight enough to keep up with me on the bottom. Her full-length keel was designed for straight towing, not turning, and needed to be reduced in size.

Once a big swell set in, I had her hauled out, and I cut about a ton of deadwood from her keel, eliminating the turning problem. Her boxy house and mechanical steering arrangement required iron determination. This contraption constructed with pulleys and cables appeared to be as ancient as that on a square-rigger.

After two additional weeks of good diving, another large swell provided me with the opportunity to rebuild her steering and construct a new house.

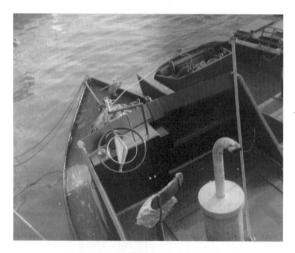

ROSY STEERING WHEEL

70

I never enjoyed marine steering controls; normally, they are a disaster to install and use, so I visited an auto wrecker and bought an entire 1951 Ford steering system — gear box, pitman arm, steering column, and wheel. I mounted the entire arrangement through the roof of my new house and ran a push-pull pipe under everything and to the rudder's tiller. We could then steer the old barge with one finger.

Her rebuilt house now had decent accommodations forward and, after a coat of black paint, my guano barge even <u>looked</u> good. I completed all of this in two weeks, just in time for the return of good weather. Now we had no excuses. We could go after abalone with a vengeance and (maybe) keep up with Don Gallagher and Ed Wood. On the other hand, that might be pushing things.

I didn't realize the 1939 Buick engine was living on borrowed time; I didn't know it had been removed from a wrecked hay rake on a local ranch five years earlier. And soon the mill started acting up, farting and coughing. I pulled off the intake manifold — its gasket was sucked in. After installing a new one, she ran like a top. Two days later the auto engine sucked in another gasket and the farting resumed.

I eventually had the manifold milled flat; I was sure this would cure the problem, but the gasket continued to suck itself into the engine block. We would then head for home with an engine that sounded as if its ignition system had been submerged in seawater. Sometimes we barely made it back.

Perplexed, I pulled the manifold and had it machined flat a second time. Holding it against the engine block and without the gasket, I checked the alignment between them. The damned engine block had a bow of almost a quarter inch. The engine was junk. The Montgomery clan and George Veramonte had the last laugh.

The foreman at the Morro Bay Boat Works told me his boss had an engine for sale. "It's old but it ran when they replaced it. It's over there behind the shack." The little engine, a four-cylinder Hall Scott, was as cute a mill as I'd ever seen. Its bigger cousins were known for their high power. I had no idea how much poop this engine had, but it certainly looked big enough.

The boat works owner was biting off the end of a cigar as he swiveled his chair around. "The Hall Scott?" he said. "I'll take $200 for her...I'll even throw in hauling you out, hoisting the old engine out, and dropping in the little mill."

D.C. towed the *Rosy* to the boat works the next day. We put her on the ways and I cut a hole in the top of my new engine room roof. Out came the old car engine, and it was forever laid to rest in the boat works weeds. The one week I had allotted for building engine beds, aligning and bolting down the new engine, building an exhaust system, making up new controls, changing the fuel system and a new compressor mount, was not enough. And in my time line, I had completely forgotten to account for the two hundred other miscellaneous tasks ahead. The one week grew to three and, by the time *Rosy* was ready, the swell had returned. As it turned out, I needed that extra time to run out the new bugs and then clean up my mess.

I discovered my engine was a "Fisher Junior," a smaller rendition of its single, overhead cam grandfather with but twenty-five horsepower. Nevertheless, these were big ponies. Now my old barge moved through the water at almost the same speed as it had with the Buick. In all my life, I have never owned such a wonderful engine. It had duel spark plugs and a dual ignition – both a battery and a magneto that allowed me to hand-crank her if the battery was dead. This feature saved our butts several times. The Hall Scott always started on the second revolution, everything functioned, and it did not leak one drop of oil. I was in hog heaven.

Pleased as I was with the engine and its price, I was not pleased with the down time, and my bride was not pleased either. The extra two weeks had once again cost us our meager savings, and Bob's Sea Foods came to our rescue with several meals at the end of long days.

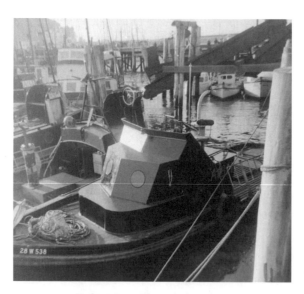

ROSY, MORRO BAY, 1957

It was now time to do some serious diving. We worked every day possible, but just as things were going well a carbuncle popped out on my knee and I was crippled for a week. Then, after a week in the water, I got another carbuncle. This one had just healed when the damn swell came up again. Then, when everything was looking good, Mel went on a binge, shacking up with Three Tit. Everytime I turned my back, it seemed another off-the-wall situation would arise. The abalone god hated me, Barney wasn't getting abalone, and our bank account was missing. On a scale of one-to-ten, I was registering perhaps two.

Oh, hell, I was registering one.

The June Gloom had long since set in. I couldn't believe how cold and wet it was at six in the morning. The foghorn blew two notes, one high and one an octave lower. To me it was moaning, "Poooor....Boooob, poooor....Boooob." I would get up in the cold mornings, climb into my wet boat in the clammy fog, only to put up with Bob's incessant laughter and stinky Mel Catrel. Unless I'd had them dry-cleaned the previous day, my wools were always damp. (They couldn't be washed because they would shrink.) Damp, they brought on another carbuncle costing me another week. Treasuring my memories of warm San Diego, I began to dwell on Santa Barbara with its tropical climate. God how I wished we were living there. One problem remained concerning the *Rosy*; there was no way of knowing when she would take on water and do her best to sink. She would stay dry for a week, then darn near go down overnight. Leaving her anchored for a weekend was like playing Russian roulette. Would I then discover only an anchor and chain attached to an oil slick?

The Black Fleet moved thirty miles north to San Simeon where we anchored in the protected San Simeon cove. An amphibious, World War II "duck" took us out to our boats but, since the taxi didn't operate on weekends, I had to swim out to the *Rosy* to check on her, and the water was extremely cold. On the days when I checked her, she hadn't taken on any water; then one day when I didn't check she came close to sinking and my prized new battery flooded. Thank God for Mr. Hall, Mr. Scott, and their engine that could be hand-cranked.

The abalone around San Simeon were thinning out and, after three months of working Beckett's Reef, it grew more and more difficult to bring in fifteen dozen. The Black Fleet then returned to Morro Bay with *Rosy* poking along in pursuit. There I ran into Laddie. He had tied up his worn-out *Pretty Babe* and was now diving Barney's *Paula*, the sister boat to the *Cathy*. "I have a great idea," I told him. "Let's run our boats south to Avila and anchor them by the pier. We'll leave early the next day and run to Purisima Point. I know there are a slug of abalone there somewhere." (Vandenberg Air Force Base is located near Purisima Point today.)

It would be a long run down and an even longer run back against the wind, so Laddie was reluctant. But he didn't want to let me down. We didn't need our crews for the run to Avila, so it would be just the two of us. The following morning I waited for him at the dock until eleven, then I decided to tow the *Paula* the fifteen miles myself. I had very limited experience, towing boats at sea, and I used a short line until both boats were in open water. Then I payed out sixty feet and opened the throttle on my Fisher Junior. The *Paula* began sheering back and forth. It was obvious she was going to part the line so I had to change plans.

I tied the two vessels together with several auto tires between. The two boats then devoured one another with every swell. I got a bright idea — I would start the *Paula*. That worked, and I soon had both boats up to speed, a foot apart and traveling like mad. The boats might have looked like a disjointed catamaran or a plywood sea monster but, tied together, they were moving faster than either boat could have moved by itself.

When I spotted the Black Fleet working behind Pecho Rock, I decided to greet Barney who was operating the *Lorraine W* for Ed Wood. I had forgotten that both boats actually belonged to him. All he could do was shake his head. "Two boats and one man, oh my God."

Barney never did like me.

Against all odds, I managed to pull into Avila with no problems. Now all I had to do was anchor the *Rosy*; the *Paula* was already tied up alongside. I got a boat ride into the pier where I ran into George the Greek who was, originally, a sponge diver from Tarpon Springs, Florida. He had hired my old friend George Rebuck as his operator and I was glad to see them both. They had been working the Avila mudflats, but the area was now picked over and, when I told them of my plan, they asked to accompany Lad and me. I was delighted.

Returning to Morro Bay, I phoned Laddie. He was simultaneously upset and relieved. He found the *Paula* missing and had forgotten about my scheme. Now he was committed to make the run south — a run he had never intended to make in the first place. Friendships often come with baggage!

The next day our three boats left Avila at five and, when the sun came up, we were promised a beautiful day. Five hours later, reaching our destination, we eased into the kelp beds. By noon, none of us had any abalone. By four we had a couple. All eyes were now on me, and I didn't blame them. We had made the long trip for nothing, and the trip home would be even longer; longer, colder, and without a hot meal. Our friendship would be strained. "Oh well," I told myself, "sometimes, even when your intentions are good and you do your best, you lose." This seemed to be one of those times.

By five in the evening we decided to head north while licking our wounds. Then, before dressing out, I jumped a single strand of kelp that was further offshore and, when I landed on the bottom, I discovered abalone everywhere — on top of one another and all around me. I was surrounded by abalone, and they were huge. Some were even too large to fit through the bag ring. What a sight!

After quickly filling a bag I called for a second, and I had it filled before the previous bag had been pulled up on deck. Laughing Bob was not laughing; he was in a panic. "We don't have another bag," he told me. "You'll have to wait." While waiting, I stacked abalone so I could roll them into an empty bag quickly. "Bob," I told him, "Don't measure any. Just dump the bags on deck."

In half an hour, I had picked the virgin spot clean. Then I made a wide circle. There were no abalone left. When I came up, Lad's boat was very close. His tender was dumping bags of abalone on top of his stack, and they were rolling down and back into the water so Lad would have to re-bag them.

The Greek was doing the same thing.

Later, when the three of us were standing on our ladders, we looked at one another and held our hands to the sky. "Thank you God!"

Landing in what may have been the last virgin bed on the coast, we had won our gamble. I had thirty-five dozen, Lad had fifty, and the Greek had forty. Back home we received twice the usual price for the monsters.

The return trip home was not an easy one, however. Because the *Rosy* was now painted black, her planks were heated by the sun, drying out her seams above the waterline. Because our load of abalone was so large, the opened seams were being pushed under water. In spite of her large bilge pump, the *Rosy* was sinking. I leaped into the engine room and frantically began bailing out the now-flooded cement bathtub. The water came in as fast as I bailed. The *Rosy* was doomed unless I tossed the abalone overboard or pulled a rabbit from my hat. Losing the abalone was out of the question — my only other option was to throw Mel overboard, and I considered it.

Then the abalone god came to my (and Mel's) aid. He told me to remove the engine's water intake hose, close the sea cock, and let the Fisher Junior's cooling pump assist in removing the sea water. This worked.

The other boats had their hands full as well. The deck on the *Paula* was huge and overloaded, rendering her unstable. The crew threw enough of the mollusks into the engine room to uncover the rear hatch, and then they filled the hold. The Greek and George Rebuck were having to do the same thing.

We arrived back at the Avila Pier around midnight, then stayed aboard our boats and pumped until morning. Barney drove his old ton-and-a-half Studebaker shell truck onto the pier, and we unloaded the *Rosy* and *Paula* into it. The truck was so full it could barely move, so we made the trip to Morro Bay at twenty-five miles an hour. The Greek was working for Harold Elmore. He sent a pickup which made two trips.

At the plant, our stack of abalone was absolutely enormous. The Black Fleet divers who came to look at it went away jealous. A first for me.

In spite of the many raised eyebrows, I grew to not only tolerate the old barge but to love her. At the end of the summer, Claudia and I decided to move to Santa Barbara, setting off Barney's Irish temper. I told him I would put the *Rosy* up for sale and eventually pay him back. The *Rosy* remained anchored in Santa Barbara, awaiting a buyer. She would never again see the Channel Islands, have a diver on her ladder, or have her deck filled with abalone.

A Polish gentleman eventually purchased her. He had never before been on the ocean and knew nothing about fishing or the mechanics of running a boat, but he just had to have her. After a run around the harbor, he was hooked. He loved her, wrote me a check for $2000, and I was able to repay Barney. I kept her diving gear and gave it to Laddie who desperately needed my helmet which, by then, had an enlarged, rectangular faceplate.

One day a large fishing boat arrived to tow the *Rosy* to Ventura. Her new owner didn't know how to start her, run her, or even pull up her anchor. On the trip south, her seams opened again, and this time there was no one aboard to pump her. Somewhere between Santa Barbara and Ventura − in approximately two hundred feet of water − there lies a steering column from a fifty-one Ford and the finest engine known to seamen, the little Hall Scott Fisher Junior. Somewhere out there, as well, is my broken heart. The truth is, *Rosy* was my clone.

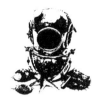

BARNACLE JIM PENN

While I was re-powering the *Rosy*, "Captain" Jim Penn and his tender, whose name I never learned, arrived from Kansas and showed up at the boat works. Both men were as salty looking as possible. It appeared as if they had read everything pertaining to the ocean, and then dressed and acted the part – as if they had sailed on a square-rigger with their dory.

Jim, with his robust body and dark features, was tall and extremely handsome. He was wearing a cobalt blue, turtleneck sweater under an unbuttoned, blue denim shirt. His black trousers were cut like those worn by east coast seaman in the days of the early sailing ships. His skipper's hat showed wear; it had been purchased from an antique store or, if purchased new, he had distressed it by beating it with a rusty chain.

He would have been a perfect stand-in for Gregory Peck in Peck's portrayal of Captain Ahab – a dapper, turn-of-the-century, down east seaman, knife and all. His tender was dressed just like Jim, only he was wearing a blue stocking cap. Determining which man was the captain was not difficult.

The members of the abalone troops, on the other hand, appeared to be ordinary working people. Unless they were attempting to impress a lady by bragging about their diving skills, you couldn't have guessed their occupation. Top abalone divers are focused and share a determination to be the best at what they do. This never changed, even as they aged. It must have born in them. Me? Well, I possessed this trait to a somewhat lesser degree. My poor abalone harvest was proof of this.

Jim Penn didn't possess one ounce of this god-given determination. Not one small piece. If he had been as good a diver as he was an actor, he would have out-picked us all. "Watch out for Captain Jim. He's a sleeper. Soon he'll be a top diver." Ha ha. Whenever I visited the Circle Inn after a hard day rebuilding the *Rosy*, I was asked to fill in the troops. How was Jim progressing with the refitting of his vessel? My report was usually good for a couple of drinks.

His boat gave him away, for a dory is inadequate for abalone diving. His only reason for being in Morro Bay was to become an abalone diver look-alike. He would return home a hero; the actual taking of abalone was not important. Acting the part was his only goal.

As I got to know him better, I learned he had been raised on a farm just outside a Kansas town. Farmers and fishermen need to be decent mechanics, and a background in farming would be very useful to someone interesting in commercial fishing. Jim was no exception; he was handy with tools.

Jim and his partner addressed one another with "matey," and assumed fey salty terms such as "aye, aye"; even their walks were affected.

All of their tools were old and hand-operated; some were even handmade. As a result, it took them far longer than it should have to install an inboard engine or diving equipment. Even more interesting, they didn't have a clue what they were doing. If it hadn't been for the yard foreman, I doubt the farmers would have ever launched their large skiff.

This adventure was to be their first on the water; they saw the ocean for the first time on a whirlwind, two-day trip to Maine where they had located and then purchased the dory. Their entire knowledge of the ocean resulted from that single trip plus some library research. Understanding this, I would have expected them to hound us with questions. I assume their pride kept them from bothering us. Perhaps they understood that sea captains don't ask; they tell.

Penn plodded through one mistake after another. His main engine, a five-horsepower, air-cooled Wisconsin with a stock short exhaust, filled his boat with toxic fumes. Once the boat was underway, the heads of the crew were forced over the side in search of fresh air. The drive shaft and propeller were bolted directly to the undersized engine's output flange; no clutch − neutral, or reverse. After they started the thing using a rope, they were on their way! If their bow wasn't aimed in the right direction, we would hear a loud, "Oh my God!" as they bounced off objects...such as other boats.

Their compressor was powered by a similar engine. Luckily, they eventually wised up and added a large diameter intake hose that could be secured upwind, or we would have had a dead farmer and a leaderless tender on our hands.

The compressor and a Widolf mask were the only pieces of decent equipment they owned; the rest was a screwed together, non-seagoing assemblage of hardware and wood. The ocean must have appeared very forgiving when imagined from a Kansas cornfield.

Once their package was complete, Penn nailed a large hawser around the dory's gunwale so as to appear very salty. They were then ready for a sea trial.

Captain Penn sat in the narrow stern, holding the pipe tiller under his armpit while his tender started the Wisconsin. Once underway, they headed downwind into the protected shallow and flat bay − hardly an acid sea test. Later, running against an ocean wind chop, they discovered their dory made only two or three knots. Our one-hour run to the radar station took them three, and they arrived soaking wet.

Penn solved this problem by donning his wet suit before departure; his tender wore foul-weather gear. The spark plugs of both the main engine and the diving compressor were regularly shorted out by saltwater spray, and our Kansas seamen then drifted until they could be towed − usually by one of Harold Elmore's boats. Harold had been sweet-talked into funding their adventure — something none of us could understand as Harold was a seasoned diver and seaman. But then, Penn had a silver tongue.

The days went by. No abalone found its way into Jim Penn's boat. Even the worst divers found some mollusks, but Captain Jim had not one to show for his days of labor, searching the ocean's floor.

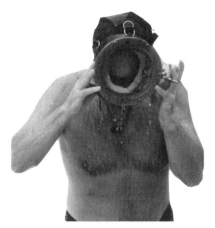

JIM PENN

When the Black Fleet ran to San Simeon to work Beckett's Reef, Penn talked someone into towing him there. Our boats anchored in San Simeon Cove and our Kansas farmers were now provided with an advantage. They didn't need to be towed for local diving because the nearby reefs were a smorgasbord of shellfish. Failing to find abalone was an impossibility.

On our runs in, the *Lorraine W* passed the dory everyday. Ed normally had twenty dozen abalone on deck; even a klutz like myself had acquired fifteen. But Penn took no shellfish — absolutely none — and he had worked hard all day. Dive after dive produced only empty bags.

Ed Wood grew tired of this. One noon break, Barney tied the *Lorraine W* alongside the salty dory, and Ed told Penn to follow him down. Both men landed on top of several abalones. Ed pointed at one. Penn shook his head in disapproval. Then Ed grabbed Penn's hand, shoved his abalone bar under the mollusk, then handed the abalone to Penn who responded by shaking his head back and forth. An angry Ed returned to his ladder.

When Penn surfaced and removed his Widolf mask, Ed shouted at him. "What the hell's the matter with you? I took an abalone off a rock and gave it to you! What more do you need?"

"I couldn't take it," Penn told him. "It had barnacles all over its shell, and I only take clean abalone. I'm Captain Jim Penn with a family tradition to uphold. We Penns are pure people. Tarnished abalone won't do. I need clean ones."

Next time a swell came in the entire Black Fleet was at the Circle Inn, laughing about the incident, when who should walk in but our salty team. Instead of his captain's hat, Jim Penn was now wearing a dark blue stocking cap. He shook all our hands as he walked around. "Thanks guys," he said. "You have been good to us. The truth is, I'll never be an abalone diver. We're going to take Ed's advice and go back to farming."

Then the two of them walked out and we never saw them again. It felt strange. Suddenly, Jim Penn was no longer the butt of our jokes. We sat on our stools, staring at the floor. Then I broke the ice. "Maybe we should have helped them more..."

I was cut off by Ed. "Look guys," he said, "Penn is not an abalone diver. But he is a winner. He'll return to Galt and tell sea stories for years. I can almost hear him saying, 'There we were in Morro Bay. We built an abalone boat and then dove it. We worked Beckett's Reef and saw more abalone than there are seashells in Mexico. We were friends with the best divers on the coast and used to get drunk with them. Then one day we got homesick, so we came back.'"

Ralph Eder's head was, as usual, on the bar. He lifted it and recited his familiar ditty. "We don't drink. We don't chew. We don't go with girls who do."

The rest of us joined in for the chorus. "Our class won the Bible."

For years, the old east coast dory lay in the weeds alongside the ramshackle office at the boat works. Then it disappeared.

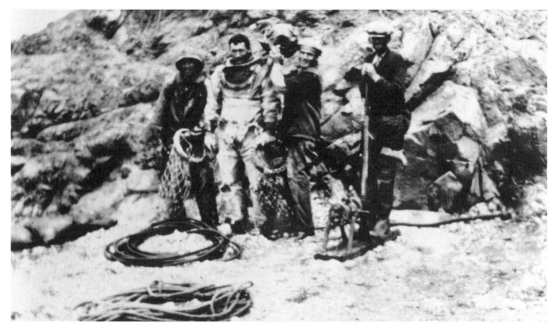

Scrap Lundy
BILL PIERCE AND CREW SHORE-PICKING

Bill Pierce founded the Morro Bay abalone fishery in 1926 when he began "shore picking" at low tide. At this time the mollusks were either exposed or just under the water, and his hunting grounds ran from Morro Bay to Ragged Point, approximately fifty miles north. Bill sought sites where the road lies close to the beach, allowing easy access.

A couple years later, using heavy gear, Pierce began diving from the shore. His gear consisted of an old navy diving helmet and a 1911 hand-operated air-compressor, both built by the Schraeder Diving Equipment Company for shallow harbor salvage work.

After observing Japanese divers from Monterey working from boats, he bought a similar craft and, following their example, upgraded his diving equipment to include their gear.

In the 1930s, while Pierce and several of his brothers were gathering large loads, Jim Beckett was making a good living shore-picking just north of the Piedras Blancas Lighthouse. Incredible tales of large, firm, red abalone with white meat filtered south to Morro Bay. Apparently, Beckett's Reef (which had by then assumed Jim Beckett's name) held enormous quantities of abalone that were piled on top of one another and sometimes lay three-mollusks deep.

When the Pierce brothers took their boats north to investigate this reef, they found an uneven rock plateau paralleling the coast north of the lighthouse for about a mile and extending perhaps half-a-mile from shore before the water became too deep to dive. The reef's bottom was indeed layered with abalone. Vertical faces were covered, and abalone were attached to rocks and hanging upside down. Because the bottom was clean and sand-free, visibility was good, even in a swell. Divers, however, had to avoid being swept along the ocean floor by the usually fierce surge.

I had heard many stories about this mecca which, it was said, contained so many shellfish a blind man could get a load. By 1957, however, most of them were not legal, and we were required to measure, then measure again. For a talented and motivated diver, a good day's work might result in perhaps twenty dozen.

It is not easy to measure abalone. If you attempt it while the mollusk is clinging to its rock, it holds fast by sucking down so securely it is difficult to remove it without damaging the meat or killing the creature. Consequently, it must be removed before it senses danger. Once removed, it is easily measured, but if it is too small it must be placed back. Unfortunately, in order for an abalone removed from a vertical or overhead surface to find a new home, it has to be set on the floor of the sea. Here it becomes vulnerable to other sea life loving the taste of the abalone's delicate white meat.

My first dive on Beckett's Reef is the one dive I treasure most. The day was warm and minus wind, and the swell was very mild with little movement on the bottom. The *Rosy* was running like a top and Mel, Bob and I were getting along particularly well. Though the water was forty-feet deep, it was so clear I could see the bottom from our boat.

Floating on the surface with the bag in my left hand and my bar in the right, I saw abalone everywhere; dark mounds only slightly camouflaged by the shifting kaleidoscope of colors. I would be rich by the end of the day.

Once I started measuring, my expectations were reined in. Almost all were shorts. Because an object appears much larger under water, I had been deceived. I continued to be overwhelmed, however, by observing the thousands of abalone covering the rocks. I kept reminding myself they were mostly shorts but, unable to convince myself, I would measure them anyway, retaining one in ten or, perhaps, only one in twenty.

I was surprised to come upon a World War I destroyer escort that had probably hit Ship Rock in the 1930s. It was recognizable because its long hull was still intact. The entire length of the hull was covered with abalone, but when I measured them I found only a few legals. Not wanting to believe my ab iron, I measured each a second time.

We were faced with this fascinating and frustrating trance all during the three months we worked Beckett's Reef. We couldn't wait to reach the bottom and, once there, we hated to come up. The water was so cold my lips would turn blue; still, I would continue my search for one small virgin area. None existed. They had all been worked over by other divers, eager as I to make a living.

It takes an abalone seven years to mature from embryo to legal size, and the steady surge of cool, clean water and abundant food at Beckett's Reef provided the perfect conditions for the nurturing of this vast population. Our whirling propeller blades yielded a bonus by cutting up and blending the bull kelp which is the abalone's most important food. The more we worked, the faster the mollusks grew.

Most members of the Black Fleet worked here in the late summer. I had the *Rosy*, Ed Wood dove the *Lorraine W,* Ralph Eder dove the *Whirlaway*, Don Gallagher the *Cathy*, Frank Briceno dove the *Paula*, and George Mitchell dove Barney's smallest boat, the *Nina.* D.C. Todd dove Jerry's *Sea Deuce*, and Laddie had his weathered *Pretty Babe* — that is, whenever she could make it from Morro Bay and Bill Seabright was sober enough to head in the right direction.

When an operator or diver was too sick to work, we filled in for one another. One day Barney had a bad cold and could not operate for Ed Wood. I took his place because Mel was shacked up with Three Tit and, since Seabright was on a toot, Laughing Bob operated for Laddie. By continuing to spell one another while working for good divers, we were all rewarded handsomely. Working with the Black Fleet was lots of fun.

One day when I was operating for Ed Wood, we were surprised by a "sneaker." A sneaker is a large, fast-moving rogue wave, probably the result of a small sea-quake, that builds to an enormous size as it passes over a shallow bottom. Ed was on his ladder with his helmet removed when the granddaddy appeared, and he yelled at me to hit the throttle so that we could climb the wall of water and keep the *Lorraine W* under control.

We had been diving at about thirty feet, and the wall we climbed was fifteen- or twenty-feet high. Once on top, I looked down forty-five feet at exposed rocks and three-foot-high palm kelp on the sea floor. My heart stopped.

I pulled back on the power, and we slid into the abyss. I was afraid our boat would strike the ocean floor where it would either founder or be broken in two pieces. Ed, wearing heavy gear and minus his helmet, would be lost.

Instead, the bow of the *Lorraine W* lifted, and we started up the other side of the trough. Giving it all the power we had, we were once again on top. I was terribly shaken, as was Ed. I'll never forget the fear in his voice. "Good grief, Kirby. That was close." Forty-five years have passed since that incident, and I still shudder to think of it. If Mel's gonads hadn't sent him after his girlfriend and I had been on the *Rosy*, her small engine could not have pulled us up the steep bank of water, and our names would be on the list of men lost at sea in Morro Bay. My wife would have been a widow, and our two children would have never been born. It is no wonder Ed and I never again spoke of it. Being a diver can make you very humble.

Palm kelp — three-feet-high trees of kelp that look like miniature palms — were everywhere at Beckett's Reef. Bull kelp, a long, single, whip-like stalk with a flotation ball on top, is also plentiful. It is much easier to operate a boat in bull kelp than in the much thicker canopy of pea kelp that thrives in California's southern waters. In any case, the tender must use a kelp knife on a ten-foot pole to cut this marine vegetation, allowing the diver's hose freedom to move. In the old days the cutting edge was a standard scythe, like those used to cut weeds. All too often, the diver's hose would also be cut, occasionally clear through. An improved kelp knife with an opening large enough for the kelp stalk but too small for the hose was a wonderful invention. Used by all the live-boaters, it saved many lives.

The "squeeze" is a diver's worst fear. It occurs when his air hose is cut or blown out, and the helmet's non-return valve fails. Non-return valves require diligent maintainance; dirt or rubber shreds from new fittings can lock the valve open, rendering it useless.

Seawater pressure is equal to almost one-half pound (actually .445) per foot of depth. At sixty feet, this equates to a bottom pressure of a little over twenty-six pounds for every square inch of exposed area.

If a diver's average upper torso is fourteen inches in diameter, the total torso area will be around 153 square inches exposed to the seawater. This area multiplied by the bottom pressure — which is twenty-six pounds at sixty feet — equals 4000 pounds of pressure that could shove the diver up into his helmet if his hose was cut or parted on the surface.

In very shallow water, there is only enough pressure to burst the blood vessels in the diver's brain; in deeper water the pressure causes the esophagus and stomach to invert out and through the mouth — similar to a deep-water fish that has been quickly brought to the surface. Because of this grim threat, divers are encouraged to carefully maintain their non-return valves.

Frank Briceno was diving the *Paula* at Beckett's Reef. His operator was in bed with a cold and Frank mistakenly hired drunken Bill Seabright. Bill allowed the little Spaniard's hose to get into the propeller, and it was cut. Because Frank had not developed the habit of checking his non-return valve, it stayed open and he was squeezed to death. His innards were reversed through his mouth and, in convulsions, he chewed some of his stomach into pieces.

A week later Laddie was given the *Paula* to dive. He had donned Frank's hot canvas diving dress before he realized some decomposed portions of Frank were still inside. Lad threw up for the next half-hour and, for a long time, he refused to discuss the incident.

By that time, every diver who live-boated in heavy gear was using a "bail-out" bottle — a small, high-pressure air tank attached to his leather belt, with a hose running to a fitting on the breastplate. If his surface air was cut off, the diver could reach down and crack the bottle's valve, thereby releasing enough air to blow him to the surface where, hopefully, he would be picked up by his crew. If his crew was on the ball, that is.

While sitting in the Circle Inn one evening, Ed was asked, "What are the most dangerous creatures you have ever encountered in the ocean?"

Without hesitation Ed replied, "My crew."

The season continued until every abalone at Beckett's Reef had been measured and all the legals had been taken. A year would pass before a new crop would be big enough to harvest. We stayed another week before migrating back to Morro Bay, but George Mitchell decided to run the *Nina* as far north as Ragged Point while prospecting for abalone along the way. He returned to Morro Bay to report that, north of Beckett's Reef, all the abalone were dead or gone. Every one. None of us believed him. We had just returned from Beckett's Reef where thousands and thousands of abalone remained.

A couple of years later stories began to reach Morro Bay and Santa Barbara. Only a ghost population remained on the once-rich rock plateau. As a result of a protection policy passed fifty years earlier, the sea otter population had been steadily increasing. After depleting the Monterey area, they had expanded south, plundering all shellfish in their path. Sea otters consume one-third of their own weight each day, and cannot exist on a smaller diet. Once the abalone are gone, they will eat all other shellfish, including starfish and sea cucumbers.

But abalone is their prime food and, since they don't know the difference between those that are legal and those that are too small, they turn over rocks and devour the babies. Soon, all the abalone were gone – there were none north of Morro Bay. A few years later as the otters migrated further south, they reached Point Conception. Along the way they decimated their favorite food and most other shellfish as well, leaving the rocks barren.

I still find it hard to visualize Beckett's Reef minus its rich and wonderful sea life. In 1994, Claudia and I camped at a spot overlooking this reef and the lighthouse. I attempted to fish off the rocks, but I never saw a single fish, let alone catch one. No more starfish were clinging to the rocks; no shellfish at all. Just sea anemones, rocks, and seaweed.

The tidal zone seemed stripped of most living creatures. At any time, otters could be seen offshore, eating something. The sea life they are consuming require time to grow, so it is not difficult to imagine the eventual fate of the otters as well. They will starve to death once they finish devouring their food chain.

Several years ago our less-than-knowledgeable California Department of Fish and

Game was determined to save some of the now-starving otters. After a long and heated dispute with the commercial fishermen of Santa Barbara, they transferred a herd of otters to San Nicholas Island — too far offshore for the otters to reach by swimming on their own. San Nick was still home to a large abalone population at the time but, two years later, all were gone and the sea otters had starved as well.

In 1951 and during my year as a lab assistant with the fish and game biology department at Stanford University, I asked Mr. Fry, our head biologist, what was going to happen to the information we were accruing during our studies. When would we turn this information over to the fish cops and ask them to enact laws based on our findings?

Mr. Fry was a giant of a man and, swiveling around in the large office chair (broken by his weight) he told me they would never use our material. He informed me there was no connection between the fish cops and the biology department, and there never would be.

"Why are we doing these studies in the first place?" I asked. He studied the ceiling while considering my question. Then he dropped his head and, looking me straight in the eye, he said, "Because they pay us to do so."

My childhood was spent in an environment of liberals and Democrats. All of us were poor, having come from the New Deal side of the tracks, and my family voted and lived as Democrats. But after my conversation with Mr. Fry I became a conservative, and a staunch conservative at that.

The fish and game cop division remains the same, putting Band-aids on festering disasters that have already taken place. Strangely enough, their own biologists have always done a great job producing information on the management of fisheries. But this information seems to fall on deaf ears. Perhaps our fish cops need hearing aids.

The sea otter is one of God's creatures, and I wish them no harm. Before the eighteenth-century Russian hunters captured the otters for their valuable pelts, the otters lived in balance with the abalone. As the otters were decimated, the mollusk population exploded. Then man began to harvest them. But there were still lots of abalone. This was due, in part, to some excellent laws preventing the taking of small abalone. But as the now-protected sea otters began to increase, the remaining abalone disappeared. It is that simple.

Today our southern areas, San Francisco south, are closed to the commercial fishing of the mollusk. Unfortunately, otters don't know this and they continue to fish. It's my guess they can't read. Perhaps the abalone will return once the otters starve. I fear the end of the otter is near.

Due to the stupidity of man, history has a tendency to repeat itself.

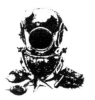

MAKE A BUCK, RIDE A DUCK, AND MR. WHITEFISH

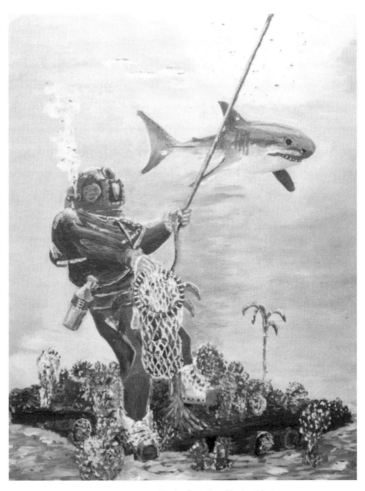

Painting by Bob Kirby

There was no pier at San Simeon, so Harold Elmore provided a surplus, WWII "duck" — an amphibious truck officially designated in 1942 DUKW — for transportation to and from our boats anchored offshore. As this over-the-hill vehicle was not a seagoing vessel, it was potentially deadly in rough water. Unloaded, the Duck had only eighteen inches freeboard. With sixty or seventy abalone on board, her ten-inch sheet metal spray rail was often the only thing that prevented her from going down.

By 1957 this veteran was at least fourteen years old. Designed to be quickly mass-produced in sheet metal, she was now riddled with holes and blobs of oxidized steel. Her only saving grace was the one-and-a-half-inch bilge pump, continuously driven off her six-cylinder gas engine.

When the Duck was running empty, the pump threw water overboard in a most-determined manner and managed to keep us afloat. Loaded, an additional number of holes were below the waterline, and the pump could not keep up with the water that was rushing in. This meant that we had around thirty or forty minutes in which to beach her before her bilges filled and we would sink.

If we were heading out to our boats in a southern swell and had to buck a rather large wave or two, we would come close to disaster. Seawater would pour through the rusty engine cover onto the distributor and either kill the engine outright or initiate a fit of uncontrolled burps and farts. Our loss of steerage in the middle of the surf would result in white knuckles and other involuntary physiological reactions.

Hector Harmony, our driver, always carried a fire extinguisher, and he would act quickly by using it to squirt a couple shots of pungent carbon tetrachloride onto the distributor cap. This displaced the seawater, and the engine would burst back to life. Thank God.

Hector was a wonderful black man who always did his best to accommodate our needs − and with a smile. My guess is, since he lived in the small town of Harmony just south of Cambria, his surname was of his own choosing and was not his legal handle. He had only one handicap − he was almost blind. We would point out our boats and guide him towards them, but he never saw their black shapes until it was too late. Collisions between the steel Duck and our wooden boats always sounded terminal. Hector was the only good thing about his decaying vessel.

Each morning we had to load fifty-gallon drums of gasoline up and into the Duck, and then onto the decks of our boats. We developed a technique for this, and two of us would pick up a drum and step from the deck of the Duck onto the deck of the boat with the drum between us. Fifty gallons of gas and a steel drum weigh over four hundred pounds together. I couldn't lift this today. Perhaps I'm getting old...

The trip out on the Duck was the best part of the most memorable day of my diving career. As I recall, the day began ugly and then got worse. Claudia had awakened in a foul mood. She had been working very hard the previous day, slinging fish and chips at Bob's Sea Foods, while I had taken the day off just to goof around. I even went into Bob's for a cup of coffee and to visit with my buddies while Claudia waited on us. She had prepared a great meal for us at home and was feeling resentful. Consequently, we had grumbled at each other all evening.

It was so foggy, wet, and cold the next morning that I couldn't force Mel to ride in the bed of the pickup. As usual, he smelled terrible and, even with Laughing Bob between us, his stench overwhelmed the cab. The thirty-mile run to San Simeon, particularly with the windows down, was an endless, frozen purgatory.

That morning San Simeon Bay, usually warmer than the surrounding countryside, was cold. The fog was thick and there was a northwesterly wind. After a wet drive through the breakers in the Duck, we arrived at the *Rosy* only to discover her bilges were full. Her battery was again submerged, so I had to crank the Hall Scott by hand. Once we were pumped out, my new Danforth anchor hung up on a rock. We finally managed to free it, but it was badly bent. Consequently, I was angry before we were underway.

This was to be our last day at Beckett's Reef. When it was over, I could drop my crew onto the Duck and head the *Rosy* south to Morro Bay. I couldn't wait to be alone on my old boat for a few hours, riding the soft whitecaps downwind and listening to the Hall Scott's muffled exhaust as I reflected on my life. I was pondering our next move. Should Claudia and I remain in Morro Bay? Or should we move south.

This particular day, like it or not (and I didn't like it), my next move would be into the stinking, clammy, diving wools, then into my cold dress and the smell of Mel's armpits. Then I would be entering the freezing water to measure abalone until I was too cold to do anymore measuring.

This was my chosen lifestyle; still, I felt like kicking myself in the butt. I wished the day was over. If only something could take place to shorten my last day on the reef. I didn't care what...just something. My wish would be granted in a way I could never have imagined and, by the end of the day, I was wishing I had never made my original wish.

I considered putting Bob down. He had been asking to work on the bottom and had been around long enough to know what not to do. Unfortunately, there was a tumor the size of an egg behind his ear, and the blood vessels running through it looked as if they were ready to burst. The tumor was situated right where Bob had to bump the exhaust valve inside my helmet to control his buoyancy. Consequently, the idea of Bob working on the bottom was out.

I resolved to use the day diving for abalone. This would not only make Barney happy but would also provide me with a few bucks. We ran to the northern end of Beckett's Reef, and I began dressing to dive in forty feet of water.

When Mel leaned over my head to tighten my rear brale nuts, his odor was so bad I almost upchucked. Once again, I chewed Bob out for not keeping Mel downwind. As I said before, I was not in a good mood.

Once on the bottom, I had a new problem. Claudia had prepared a wonderful chili dinner the previous night, I had made a pig of myself, and now the giant bubble of gas collecting in my lower intestine was demanding to be released. The foul, fermented gas made its way through my three sets of wools, surrounded my head and nose on its way to my exhaust valve, and I discovered that passing gas while wearing heavy gear can be almost deadly.

After an hour of torment, I had one full bag and another on deck, perhaps three- or four-dozen abalone. This spot seemed to have more legals than normal so I decided it must have been missed. By the end of the day, I might have twenty dozen — a good farewell gesture to Jim Beckett and his reef.

My bad mood was passing along with the gas. Hell, it was time to grow up, to be a man, to take whatever came along. Then Bob's voice came over the phones. "Kirby, there is a shark alongside. I think it is coming down your bubbles."

"Shark smark." I thought, reminding myself of my promise to become a man. "Who cares? A little shark is no big deal."

Out of curiosity, I looked up. Holy shit! The bastard was as large as a U.S. Navy submarine, armed with teeth, torpedoes, and a gray paint job!

Great white sharks are seldom seen on our coast, so I didn't know exactly what kind of shark it was. I only knew it was big. It had the girth of a fifty-gallon oil drum; perhaps it was even larger. Its teeth were a good inch-and-a-half long, and there were lots of them.

His mouth was closed — a good sign. However, when I observed the tangled maze of white, razor-sharp, serrated, triangular blades which were exposed around this mouth, I knew he was ready and able to go to work at any moment. That mouth was large enough to slice me in half, and if this happened he would be getting a mouthful of more than the red meat of a scared-to-death diver, for I had filled my pants.

His eyes were pools of black oil — there was no emotion, no sign of life — it was like looking into a black sewer pipe in a basement. I was sure, however, that this huge shark could see me quite well. Too well.

I knew little about sharks then and know only a bit more today. They are recognized as nature's undersea eating machines. They don't plan an attack; they simply attack on instinct. Grabbing a stalk of palm kelp, I held on tight. I have no idea why. When I noticed that the shark seemed particularly interested in my bubbles, I turned off my air and waited.

In a heavy suit, enough air remains to sustain a person for four minutes before panic sets in. Two minutes went by before I ventilated. I felt slightly relieved because the shark seemed to have departed. But just to make sure before reopening my air supply valve, I turned around very slowly. The big bastard was three feet behind me!

Our game of hide-and-seek continued. Mr. Whitefish would depart, then turn up again. I would hide behind the small palm kelp while he would seek me out. I have no idea how long this continued. Frightened as I had never before been in my life, I lost all track of time.

I knew that the exposed nerves running the length of each side of a shark's body can pick up the electrical currents emitted by creatures in panic and, because there was a chance my electrical telephone impulses might further arouse the killer, I did my best not to communicate with Bob.

Our game continued. The shark would leave, then return to check out my backside. One time when he didn't return, I checked in all directions. No gray submarine, so I announced to Bob that I was coming up. Repeating my command, he positioned the *Rosy* so that her ladder was alongside my bubbles. I turned on my air and held tightly onto the palm kelp. My dress filled until I was too buoyant to hold on any longer. "Coming up," I said. I came up so rapidly that I was blown five feet out of the water. Then, in one maneuver, I ended up on the ladder and the deck.

Mel removed my helmet. Neither of us spoke. I sat on my deck box for awhile, then asked Bob for a cup of coffee. He asked where I wanted to go next. "Are you kidding?" I answered. "To Morro Bay. That big bastard is going to follow the *Rosy* wherever it goes, probably even into the harbor. He wants to eat me. I won't give him another chance. We are out of here."

I dressed out, then delivered Bob and Mel to Hector on the Duck. They could drive my pickup back, and I would run the *Rosy* alone to Morro Bay as previously planned. I had just not planned to do it with a shark on my mind.

I continued to tremble for days. Since that time, I have come close to death several times during a dive, usually because of some stupid mistake on my part.

For some reason, none of these close calls disturbed me until they were over. But my experience with the shark was different. Once while working in the offshore oil patch, I sat on a decompression bar that was being jerked up and down. I felt like a human fishing plug and knew I was waiting for that shark to show up again. After my experience with the shark, I never again enjoyed construction diving unless it took place in black water where I felt I had a fighting chance to hide. And I never again enjoyed sport diving as much as I had before this encounter. I was frightened senseless from the moment the shark first appeared, and I am still frightened when I think about it today.

No matter where, when, or how I dove, I wondered if that big, gray, son-of-a-bitch was looking for me.

I'm still wondering.

BOB'S SEA FOODS

The joints of the broken-down fish dock screamed their complaints as the huge fishing boat pulled first this way, then that, moved by the fast outgoing tide that was fighting a strong, cold, northern wind. The water was boiling and turbulent. All boat lines were secured to blocks of concrete sitting against the huge rocks strewn along the bank, a necessity because the dock's cleats had long ago vanished by simply rusting away. On top of the pilings still left standing were rotting timbers and decomposed planks, sort of a walkway that required careful navigation and a life insurance policy.

The long steel boom of the rust-stained old dragger swung out, and a load of beautiful red bottom fish were dumped into an over-the-hill, two-wheeled cart. The only worker on the dock pushed this contraption through a broken door and into the rear of the dilapidated, tin-covered shed. He then slid the load onto the slimy, pot-holed, cement floor.

A muscular young man picked out a fish, cut behind the gill, made a single slice against its backbone all the way to the tail, then slid the razor-sharp knife down one side, removing the skin. This yielded a clean, fresh filet. He then turned the fish over and repeated his moves. The entire operation took perhaps five seconds.

Bob was a workout freak and weight lifter. He was thirty-four-years old and, with his Nordic features, blonde hair, and freckles — was very good-looking. He had a strong jaw, a cheerful face, and was a perfect proprietor and wonderful friend. His wife, Dotty, olive-skinned and small, was a knockout. And, like Bob, she was full of life. Dotty always viewed the glass as half-full. She and Bob seemed to be a perfect couple and had been together thirteen years.

Five years earlier, they had purchased the old processing plant for a substantial sum — $12,000 — a fair price for waterfront property in 1952. For the next three years this establishment continued to deteriorate while they struggled to make payments. Then the two of them hit upon the idea of a fish and chips restaurant, and from then on they were making enough money to begin the formidable task of rebuilding the place.

In a couple of hours, Bob could reduce a mound of fresh-caught fish sitting on his four-by-eight wooden table into a heaping mound of clean, white meat. These filets were then ready for the restaurant's deep fryer or for shipment to the hot central California city of Bakersfield where they were easily marketed from Bob's old refrigerator truck.

One didn't need directions to locate Bob and Dotty's waterfront restaurant — all you needed to do was follow your nose. The smell of fish frying was unmistakable, and the establishment itself, with its many years accumulation of fish being processed while the juices leaked on the floor and into its many cracks and seams, reeked of the sea and salt air.

Though the customers enjoyed the atmosphere, the local health inspector did not. A small man with an equally small attitude, the inspector knew the way to Bob's Sea Foods well, for he had been there many times. He was of German descent, intimidation was the name of his game and, for reasons never understood, he had apparently taken a great dislike towards them and usually gave them a ration of crap at least once a week. He always arrived with a clipboard listing complaints, and he seemed to enjoy badgering them, as if this was his duty, his recreation, and his religion.

Every week he would drive up in his stripped, gray, 1956 Plymouth adorned with government plates and pull into a parking place near the restaurant.

Barney Clancy had leased the rear of the galvanized shed for his abalone plant, and he and Bob did their best to protect one another from the health inspector. Barney needed little protection because he could be even meaner than the inspector, and the two of them had long since worked out a system of mutual respect. After a series of insults and fist-shaking, Barney — with his Irish demeanor — had gained the upper hand. Or so it seemed at the time.

As good fortune would have it, the health inspector had not spotted the shack perched on the roof of Barney's plant. If he had seen it, he would have shut down the entire place in a heartbeat. Unknown to everyone except Dotty and Bob, this was where Melvin C. Catrel lived. I've described Mel several times already so...nuff said.

The restaurant was a beehive of activity. Each evening Mel processed fifty pounds of potatoes for the deep fryer; Mel peeled potatoes in exchange for room and board. (Melvin received the best end of this deal.)

As I mentioned earlier, my bride Claudia worked here, cooking and serving. When one is employed at a restaurant, there is seldom time to "smell the roses," and Dotty worked harder than everyone. Whenever things were slow, she could sneak a cup of coffee, but after taking a sip a new set of problems would usually arise to interrupt her break.

Bob and Dotty were a most-beloved couple. Their restaurant consisted of plywood and thin paint attached to a rusty, corrugated metal structure, but everyone enjoyed the great food and the companionship offered by its friendly owners. "Bob's Sea Foods" stated the crudely painted sign tacked onto the false plywood front, and it was a meeting place for local fishermen during the day and a good place to get a meal in the evening. It was always packed.

The fish menu was the best in town, and the prices were even better. You could buy an "all you can eat" meal of fish and chips, including coffee, for seventy-five cents, and shrimp was a buck-twenty-five. As a rule, there was no charge for a cup of coffee. A poor family would sometimes show up, and the father would order one meal for himself and soon return for another plateful until his family was full. When Claudia brought this to Bob's attention he said, "Let them eat. They don't have much money."

Bob's Sea Foods was a lifesaver for Claudia and me. The work was hard but fun. Claudia loved Dotty and they became close friends. When the swell was up, I either worked on the *Rosy* or for Bob, rebuilding the decaying dock. This was my first exposure to pile driving and heavy marine construction, and I enjoyed it. Also, the coffee was great and I could bug my wife.

After several months with our new friends, an ugly situation arose. Bob became attracted to the lady who delivered fresh oysters her family was raising in the southern, muddy bay. All of us were hard-pressed to understand what it was about the "oyster lady" that excited Bob. It surely wasn't her looks, for she was quite ugly and so thin we wondered if she was suffering from AIDs. Her breasts were non-existent, she had scraggly teeth and sunken eyes, and she always wore muddy, oversized rubber boots. In a word, the oyster lady was a poop, pure and simple. Dotty, on the other hand, was witty, cute, and desirable. Consequently, she had no trouble retaliating and, within a short time, she found herself a good-looking boyfriend. The war was on.

By the time Claudia and I moved to Santa Barbara, Bob and Dotty had divorced, and Bob's Sea Foods was sold for a handsome profit. The restaurant retained its name and continued in business for the next thirty-five years. It more recently became "The Outrigger."

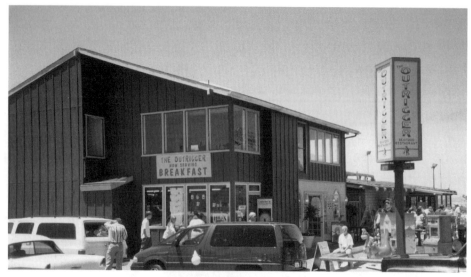

THE OUTRIGGER, 2000

For a period of time, either Bob or Dotty would stop by our Santa Barbara home for a visit. Then we sadly learned that Bob had a heart attack and died. He was only thirty-eight. Dotty soon faded from our lives as well, and Claudia and I often wonder if we'll ever learn what happened to her.

Bob and his oyster lady is a mystery that continues to mystify us. What was it that had attracted him? Perhaps it was her fish-like bodily scent. Sex is a most complex force.

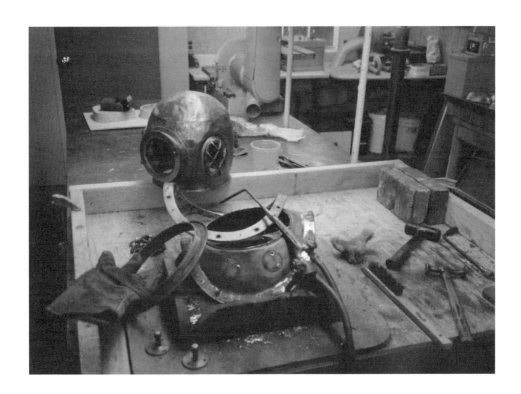

THE DIRTIEST MAN IN MORRO BAY

A dismal-looking man stared back at me from the mirror. We had been diving for two straight weeks with no reprieve granted by bad weather. I was tired of the fog, tired of Bob's irritating laugh, and tired of scroungy little Mel's never-ending, awful stink. A thirty-foot boat is not large enough to allow much separation between seamen, and the small things begin to bug you — a constant sniffle or cough, a lack of personality or too much personality, pretending to enjoy a man whom you detest. "Oh Lord, the sea is so vast and my boat is so small. Once I get ashore, I promise to head to the desert and never return."

Abalone boat operators need to keep their boats in proper position and Laughing Bob was aces until I was back on the ladder; then he would let down his guard. My one requirement was for him to keep Mel downwind. Why he couldn't follow this order was a mystery to me.

Once I was up, Bob would remove his hands from the controls, laugh, and then do a silly little dance. I imagine he was hoping to raise my spirits. It didn't work.

Mel smelled worse than a septic tank. His once-tan leather coat was now a mottled, black and dark brown, and salty stains ran from under his arms to his waist. His Levis would have stood upright if he ever removed them. I wondered how he could pull them low enough to use the can. Perhaps he never tried; instead, he just shook a leg and slung a turd or two into the water.

Mel did have some standards. He always wore white socks (I believe this was their original color) and, once they were reduced to rings around his ankles, he would remove a shoe (I hope no one was present) and pull on a new sock. The remainder of the old sock would then vanish, becoming a pungent cloud.

Every living creature has a mother, and I wondered what kind of woman had borne Mel Cornelius Catrel. Was she normal? I doubt it. Was she clean? Educated? Who knows. Melvin once admitted to having a third grade education. He had little else to say, and I didn't pursue the subject. Truth was — I could have cared less.

One night after his restaurant was closed for the night and we were drinking Scotch, Bob confessed that his potato peeler occupied the crude board and batten shack perched over the rear of the ab plant's roof. I struggled to imagine the structure's interior condition.

I hated putting on my wools. Even when they had been cleaned the previous day, they were damp and smelled almost as bad as my tender. Once they were on, I was forced to having Mel dress me in. When he leaned over to tighten my rear brale nuts, I had to hold my breath for a long time.

Once in the water, Mel was very competent. A tender is not required to possess a PhD; he is merely required to keep his head out of his butt while at sea.

We worked the radar station and ended up with my usual fifteen dozen. The *Rosy* was running well on our run in, Bob's infernal laughter had wound down and he had stopped doing his damned dance, and Melvin was situated on the bow, downwind, as I had commanded. I was enjoying a cup of warm coffee and looking forward to Claudia and my dinner date with Bob and Dotty.

Once we entered the channel, Mel jumped to his feet and landed up in the bridge with Bob and I. We had no idea why. Then, when I saw Bob's Sea Foods I could tell the little shack and portions of the tin roof over Bob's processing plant were missing. Mel had jumped up on the bridge to get a better view. His home had been destroyed and was lying in the parking lot; the remains were bound to the end of a long length of rusty cable attached to Barney's Studebaker shell truck.

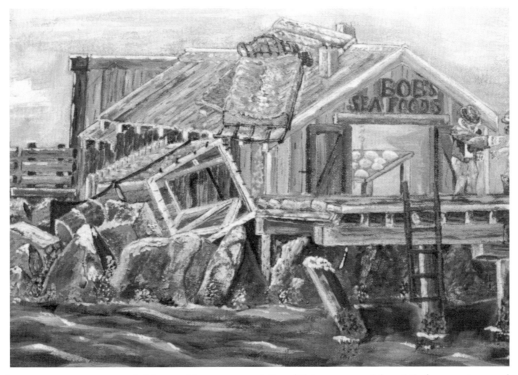

As we drew nearer we could hear Barney and the ill-tempered health inspector going at it. They were using adjectives from the devil himself. Then the processor and the health inspector began to deliver a vicious verbal attack on Bob. As we were about to tie up, Mel made a narrow escape – for many feet (and hands) were now in hot pursuit. He eventually reached the highway where he flagged down a car, headed north, and no doubt ended up in the comforting arms of his lover, Three Tit. I never saw Melvin C. Catrel again.

The story unfolded. Mel's penthouse contained no sanitary facilities, and he had been using a gallon can as a urinal. The can had long-since rusted out and its acidic contents had attacked the galvanized roof over Barney's operation. The fluid eventually ate through the steel roof and was dripping on the large table where Barney's sliced abalone were drying before being pounded.

Someone had called the county health department and the inspector had arrived with his clipboard. Then the little German began tearing into Bob and Barney.

Bob sought instant restitution, at least in part, by commandeering Barney's old truck and pulling the shack off the roof. Pieces of the roof and the room, its contents, the pee can, and what was left of the pungent interior were scattered about. I spotted Mel's mattress; its center had rotted away with urine.

Our dinner date was now cancelled, for Bob had a more important matter to attend to — how to stay out of jail.

Barney's face remained beet red for days; the health inspector with his clipboard was a constant threat. Dotty wasn't speaking to Bob and, for some reason, Bob was mad at Barney. Was it because Barney had wanted his roof repaired?

A couple of months after Claudia and I had departed for warmer waters, Bob ran into Mel in Happy Jack's and came close to terminating Mel's life. Mel's saving grace might have been the fact that he smelled so bad Bob wouldn't touch him.

Several years later I heard that Melvin Cornelius Catrel had passed out for the last time in the Circle Inn, joining Captain Jet in the big tavern in the sky.

I admit to feeling saddened by the news, but I have no idea why.

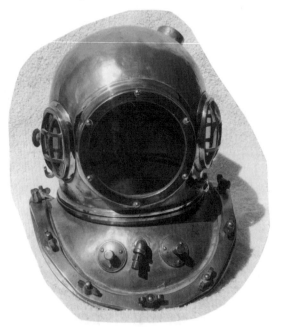

BLACK FLEET HELMET

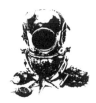

THE MAN IN GREEN

Being Jerry Todd's best friend was not easy, for I was also involved in upholding a certain legacy — his never-ending battle with the fish cops. In order to continue our relationship, I felt it was fitting — and necessary — for me to do the same.

As I mentioned earlier, short beds are a problem — for the undersized abalone as well as for myself. As a fifth-generation Californian, I felt it was my duty to assist in the elimination of both problem areas. The fish and game couldn't do it all. When it came to the management of abalone, they needed my help. Who could be better suited than me, Bob Kirby, with my guano barge and the assistance of the dirtiest man in Morro Bay and Laughing Bob? Here was a down-to-earth, flag-waving team if there ever was one.

The legal problems continued. It was illegal to take the poor, undernourished critters, so I had to come up with a new way to take them while avoiding the slammer.

Our latest warden was fresh to the fish and game; a dapper individual and a perfect ass, if there ever was one. He was the model of perfection in his uniform — no wrinkles, no stains — and it appeared as if his shoes had never seen dust, dirt, or mud. (This was probably because he always sent his assistant to do the dirty work.) My evil nature conjured up the perfect plan; I would kiss it up to him.

Everyday as the Black Fleet arrived back on the dock by Bob's Sea Foods, the warden was standing there with his assistant (fish and game logos over their black hearts), waiting for us. They measured every load, always assuming we had something to hide. To my knowledge, they never came upon a single short. Still, they persisted. Not a day passed without his presence and that of his buddy, both in their one-piece suits.

I began my scheme by filling him with bullshit. "You know," I told him one day, "I was with the fish and game myself. Always wanted to be a fish cop but had no idea how to become one. Perhaps you can help me."

After listening to my bull for a month, he offered to assist with my application as a warden.

The following day, after alerting Bob and Mel to my plan, we took off for a large short bed just south of the radar station. With the fog assisting, we raked in the abalone, shucked them, placed the few legals we had on deck, and stored the rest in sacks in the engine room. Then we met the Black Fleet at the radar station.

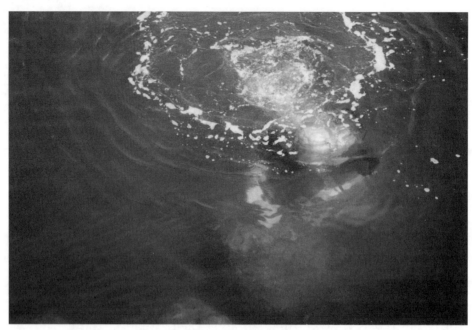

IN SHALLOW WATER

Rosy was the slowest boat in the fleet — this was the most beautiful part of my plan. Though we left with the fleet in the morning, we would always end up at the fishing grounds half an hour later than the other boats. And, because Morro Bay was always socked in by fog at this time of the year, the other boats had no idea where we were or what we were up to.

The morning went just as I had planned. The Black Fleet pulled ahead of our slow little *Rosy*. We stopped at the short bed, and eventually loaded three gunny sacks with shucked out short meat. I hid all of it on the opposite side of the engine, under a stack of hardware, rope, tools, the anchor, and our life jackets.

Once loaded, we had perhaps three dozen legal abalone on deck, enough to act as decoys for the other boats. (Actually, we produced a rather decent legal load this particularly day — maybe thirteen dozen by the time the black boats were heading home.)

The under-powered *Rosy* arrived after the rest of the Black Fleet were tied to Barney's dock. We tied up to the last boat and awaited our turn to unload.

As his helper measured the abalone — every single one — the warden kept a close watch. Now it was our turn and, I must admit, I was feeling apprehensive as we tossed our lines onto Barney's dock.

If the engine hatch was in place, I knew the turd in the one-piece suit would want to peek in, so I had instructed my team to leave the hatch cover off.

"Okay," the assistant shouted. "One more boat to measure."

"Don't bother," the warden replied. "Kirby's a good guy."

THE *PAULA*

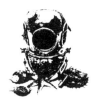

Like me, George Veramonte set out to be a lifetime, abalone diver. When he began diving around 1950, processed abalone was low in price; however, there was an abundance, and a decent abalone diver could do better diving than he could working an eight-to-five job on the beach.

After spending a couple of years diving from the old-style Japanese live boats such as the *Mollusk*, George designed the ideal abalone boat. The flying bridge was set forward and mounted on top of a low, rectangular house with a sloping front. Berths were located within the house along with a reliable marine engine fitted with a commercial, power take-off to drive the compressor. The stern's hold could accommodate large loads while smaller day loads could be stored on deck. A new trend was set with this design, and Jerry Todd copied it when he built his *Sea Deuce*.

By that time most abalone boat controls had been standardized as well. A car steering wheel was mounted vertically in the flying bridge along with a broady knob attached to one spoke. Both the throttle and the reversing lever swung in the same horizontal arc – the reversing lever was the longer of the two. You pushed forward on the throttle for power and forward on the longer handle for forward. Reverse was accomplished by pulling the lever rearward; neutral being its center.

George had two identical boats constructed, the *Paula* and the *Cathy*. Both were built to his design specifications, one for his own use and the other to be resold. Determined to attend law school, he then decided to sell both boats to Veteran's Fisheries.

Consequently, Barney Clancy now owned two of the best abalone boats in existence, and he arranged for two of the finest divers to work them; Don Gallagher dove the *Cathy* and Francisco Briceno the *Paula*.

Don operated the *Cathy* until 1959 when he turned in his abalone bar for a guide badge at Hearst Castle. After Frank was killed in that terrible squeeze in 1957, Barney offered the *Paula* to Lad Handelman, and the offer was instantly accepted as Lad's *Pretty Babe* was well over-the-hill and anchored out.

With a new boat and a new operator (Bill Seabright had retired after Frank's death) Lad wanted his first day of diving to take place close to home just in case repairs were needed or problems arose. Lad chose to make his test day behind Pecho Rock, ten miles south of Morro Bay and within five miles of the harbor at Avila.

The day got off to a very bad start as he had donned Frank's dress. (As described in a previous chapter, a portion of Frank's decomposed organs had remained in the diving dress.) Laddie turned the dress inside out and scrubbed it; still nauseous, he then dressed in the wet rig.

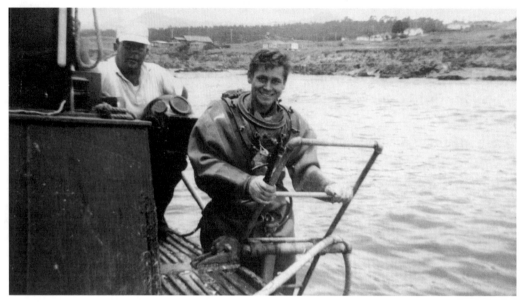

LAD ON THE *PAULA*, DRESSED IN, 1957

Despite the cold fog, the soaked wools, and diving in fifty-five-degree water, Lad did well on the bottom. Then a sneaker, somewhat like the one that had almost nailed Ed Wood and me, surprised the crew by lifting the *Paula* out of the water and impaling her on a rock. Lad came up, dressed out, and joined his men while they considered what steps to take next.

Both the crew and the boat were in a tight spot. They were alone — we didn't have radios in those days — and the tide was high so the chance of their floating free was slim. The bottom of the boat was now a sieve. If they were successful in re-floating the *Paula*, keeping water out would be difficult if not impossible. They were stranded about a hundred yards offshore, near enormous rocks and crashing breakers, and odds were against their survival if they attempted a swim to the beach.

Their least hazardous bet was to attempt to free the vessel, then patch her large holes by stuffing them with rags. They tied two life jackets to the anchor and Lad tried to swim out, but after swimming a short distance the jackets came untied and the anchor dropped. When they hauled in on the anchor chain in an attempt to move off the rock, there was insufficient holding scope, and the anchor simply came up.

They attempted this maneuver a second time with two more jackets but, because the anchor chain was so heavy, Lad couldn't swim very far and he had to cut the anchor free. Again, it wouldn't hold. Returning to the *Paula*, he was so cold he couldn't speak. As the black boat continued to swing and grind on the rock, the existing holes were enlarged and new holes appeared. Their plight grew more perilous as time passed.

Lad had but one option. Donning a life jacket, he would try to make it to shore. Then he would walk five miles south to the lighthouse, contact the coast guard, and hopefully return in time to save the lives of his two crewmen. The *Paula* was lost. This was a foregone conclusion.

Engulfed in white, crushing foam, Lad battled the breakers that were smashing against the rocks. As he struggled, he prayed.

Miraculously, he eventually reached the shore. Bruised, bleeding, and still so cold he could barely move, he staggered up a dirt road. As he plodded along like a zombie, his body temperature began to rise and his pace gradually increased. Driven by a responsibility towards his helpless crew, he pushed himself, hoping he could make the five-mile journey in an hour or, at best, an hour and a half. How could he ever tell their families that they had perished and he had survived?

A brown pickup suddenly approached from behind; "Jamansen Ranch" was printed on the its door. This would be his salvation! A ride to the lighthouse and a reprieve for his crew!

Instead, the rancher asked Lad why he was trespassing on the ranch road.

"My boat is impaled on a rock," Lad explained, "and I'm going for help. The lives of my crewmen are in grave danger."

"Turn around, go back to your boat, or I'll shoot you." Laddie couldn't believe what he was hearing. "Look," he pleaded, "I'm frozen to death, my crew is in bad shape, and my boat is wrecked. Once the owner finds this out, my life will be over anyway. Go ahead and shoot. I won't be any worse off than I am now."

The rancher turned around, drove away, and Lad resumed trudging down the dirt road. Gaining strength, he began to run and soon made the lighthouse where all hands were alerted. Lad was given a dry jacket and then driven to the fishing pier in Avila. He was very relieved to spot the coast guard boat, heading north.

Several minutes later the *Paula*, low in the water, rounded the rock jetty. The two men on board were bailing as if their lives depended on it. On the pier, Freddie Steel, the owner of the boat works, dropped the vertical ways to receive the small black abalone boat. Then, just as the *Paula* entered the welcome arms of the wooden structure, she sank. She had been caught and saved by God himself.

An incredible tale followed. A second huge breaker had lifted, then washed the *Paula*, off the rock. The desperate crewmen Lad had left behind quickly started the engine, pushed the throttle to full speed, pointed her south, and began bailing as rapidly as possible. They jumped up to the wheel only when necessary.

After hearing their story, Laddie went behind a shed and wept.

I was summoned and, the following day, Barney, Laddie, his crew, and I surveyed the damage. The *Paula's* plywood bottom looked like a dripping, shaggy dog with some pieces of wood hanging down and others protruding inward. We sawed off the wild wood, overlaid her entire bottom with plywood, and sealed the overlay with gallons of "Henry's Roofing Cement." Fred Steel installed a new strut bearing, shaft, and propeller. Three days later the *Paula* was again floating in the calm waters off Avila Bay.

Barney, who had disliked me intensely up to that time, thanked me for my efforts. Lad and I became even closer friends and have remained so through the years. The rancher, the worst kind of human, should have gone to jail.

There are laws concerning the refusal of aid to distressed seamen, and I figure he must have gone to hell after he died. When he arrived the devil asked him to choose which room he wanted to live in for eternity, and the rancher picked the room filled with beautiful ladies, each packing a bottle of Scotch. Once inside the room, the rancher noticed that each bottle had a hole in its bottom.

"This is true," the devil told him. "but the girls do not."

By the mid-sixties, with the exception of two, every one of the old-time Black Fleet heavy gear divers had changed occupation. Fast Radon boats, dead-boating, and swim gear had replaced older seamen in pursuit of the constantly decreasing abalone population.

Barney moved to Santa Barbara where he shared a building with Dutch Pierce at the end of Stearns Wharf and continued to process mollusks. (Dutch's older brother, Bill Pierce, was a Morro Bay abalone pioneer.) Then, in 1974 after working with them for two years, Barney sold out to Pierce Brothers Fisheries and retired.

Sometime in 1975 I was walking down one of the finger docks in Santa Barbara and I came across the now-forlorn little *Paula*, still painted black but missing her engine. A young hippie girl was living on the once-proud craft, and the *Paula's* diving gear had been replaced by potted plants and household items; hardly a fitting end for one of Barney's most wonderful boats. The next time I looked the *Paula* had disappeared; probably hauled off to the dump like many of her other black sisters.

The era of the Black Fleet, boats that had terrorized the ocean, was gone. Several years ago a dear friend who owns a Santa Barbara apartment complex found an old abalone helmet in the weeds after a tenant had left, and he gave it to me. I recognized it as one of the Black Fleet helmets that had probably been used aboard the *Cathy*, the *Whirlaway*, or the *Lorraine W.* After restoring it, I donated it to the Santa Barbara Maritime Museum. There, a reminder of the Black Fleet lives on forever.

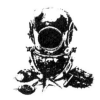

PLEASE MR. RYAN, I DON' WANNA GO

In the fall of 1957 after our move to Santa Barbara, I anchored the *Rosy* at Bradley's Reef, an underwater mound of sand that had been steadily growing since the breakwater was constructed in the 1920s. Except for an occasional spurt of activity, I gave up my career as an abalone diver. Instead, I hoped to get into oil field diving; that is, if I could persuade Jerry Todd to pull the right strings. In the meantime, I had to find a real job or we would once again starve. <u>That</u> hadn't changed.

Rosy had an extremely ugly dredge as a neighbor, a large gray box that held a couple of screaming engines and wore a sign on its side: "Ryan Construction Company." Mr. Ryan had earned his reputation as a cheap man, and his frugality was displayed by the design of his dredge.

Hank, the harbormaster, directed me to Mr. Ryan's one-room office in the low rent, veteran's memorial building across the street from his sand-eating device. A thin, graying man in his forties, Mr. Ryan was sitting in a worn office chair. He was wearing an expensive suit — I soon learned he wore fine threads even when he was forced to get down and dirty — which was not an uncommon occurrence.

"I'm Bob Kirby," I announced, "and I need a job." I held out my hand, but he didn't take it. Cold and emotionless, he seldom looked at me during the interview.

"Can you run a boat?" he asked.

"Yup."

"What else can you do?"

"I'm a welder and a diver."

"Good. I need a welder, not a diver. Walk out the pipeline to the dredge. Tell the lever man, Virgil, you are his new mate. You will have to join the operating engineers. You will get six dollars an hour; overtime is time-and-a-half."

"When do I start?"

"Right now."

I walked out the long, rock breakwater and onto the unwanted sand spit that was extending further and further each winter. It was October — days are short in October — and it was six in the evening and dark by the time I reached the twelve-inch-diameter floating pipeline. The pipeline consisted of a series of pipe sections, each perhaps twenty-five feet long, mounted on large can floats. The sections were joined by rubber couplers.

The two-by-twelve wood walkway was cold, wet, and covered with slippery sea gull guano. Jumping four feet over each joint in an effort to clear the rubber couplers was like playing Russian roulette and, just as I was nearing the dredge, the pipeline behind me broke. The resulting geyser erupted at 100 pounds per square inch, whipping both the pipe and me about like two aroused pit bulls in a fight.

I lost my footing and the bag carrying my new overalls, and my lunch ended up in the drink. I was hanging on like a rodeo cowboy, my crotch and belly now covered with stinking bird crap. Welcome to the wonderful world of dredging.

Virgil, an Oklahoma transplant, was a prince. After rescuing me he handed me a cup of coffee which he asked me to down quickly. He then told me to move the port anchor. "Y'all cain run a boat, cain't you?"

I noticed the boat, appropriately named the *Scow*, was a twenty-by-thirty-foot box constructed of rusty, rectangular WWII steel floats that had been welded together. Consequently, it had no running lines. Nothing about her construction was plumb or nice. On her bow was a huge steel A-frame. Below this tower and aft, sat a large wire winch that powered the line running through a snatch block. This was secured under the top member of the pipe framework. All I had to do was run the scow up to the anchor's crown buoy, attach the hook to the crown wire loop, engage the winch, lift the thousand-pound anchor, run it to its new location, and drop it again. A simple task.

As soon as I had the rusty monster in the windy channel, her Chrysler Royal gas engine ran out of fuel. With the A-frame serving as an excellent sail, my new commander and I beat a course directly downwind towards the Harbor House Restaurant, a large building in the center of Stearns Wharf.

I quickly tied a short piece of line — the only line on board — to a large length of welded pipe lying on the deck. Then, hopefully intending to slow our progress, I threw it over the side of the scow. My makeshift anchor came tight, then loose again. "Oh shit!" I had lost the pipe.

We continued our assault on the Harbor House, with the awkward scow weaving in the heavy, early winter swell. I had been a dredger man for maybe an hour, and it looked like I would destroy a restaurant, sink a scow, and set a new record for a career change.

The rolling steel framework struck the false eaves projecting out four feet from the restaurant. The rolling continued as the eaves were hammered into thousands of tiny pieces. Cedar shingles and chunks of four-by-fours rained on me and the scow. We soon resembled an unorganized Mexican stake-bed truck on a roofing job.

As the scenario continued, the manager and patrons of the fine eating establishment watched from a prudent distance, standing clear of the large and vulnerable plate glass window that appeared to be enjoying its last moments.

Seizing my only line, the one with which I had attempted to anchor, I tied the scow to the first pile I could reach. Grabbing the only gas can, I clambered off the scow and ran to the gas station then located at the foot of Stearns Wharf.

The owner, an ex-fisherman referred to as "Goofy Glen" Miller, gave me crap about not having money to pay for gas; then he realized I would kill for it.

I had the old Chrysler fired up and, five minutes later, I had the port anchor moved to its new position. Our deck was covered with broken shingles and, as I was rounding up the wooden debris, I looked up into the face of my new boss who was wearing a suit covered with bird shit. (Mr. Ryan was apparently no more skillful than me when it came to leaping over rubber pipe couplings.)

He was livid, and he addressed Virgil as though I wasn't there; hell...as if I wasn't even in the same county. "What happened?" he shouted.

"Well Boss," Virgil said, "the scow rain out of fuel. I guess Kirby haid to find him some gas ait Miller's station. I cain see a few shingles missin' on the restaurant, but I don't think the place got hurt none."

Still scarlet, Mr. Ryan turned to me. "Okay," he said, "put the new tailpipe on the dredge."

"I can't," I told him.

"Why the hell not?!"

"Because I threw the tailpipe overboard trying to slow the *Scow*."

Mr. Ryan turned and left, sliding in bird poop as he went. He never really liked me much after that.

The next day was a Sunday. I grabbed Claudia and we rented some scuba gear and a skiff and rowed out to where the tailpipe ought to have landed. I dropped anchor, went down its line, tied on a circling line, and started a circle search. I quickly found the pipe, tied the line to it, swam the other end to the skiff, and attached it to a small lobster buoy.

Monday, Mr. Ryan was business as usual. "Okay," he said, "weld up a new tailpipe."

I butted in with, "I will if you want, but we don't have to." His face once again turned red.

"What the hell do you mean by that?"

"See that lobster buoy?" I said, pointing. "It has your tailpipe on the other end."

"Okay. Run me into the breakwater."

I guess that was Mr. Ryan's way of saying thanks and telling me I still had a job.

Working as a mate on a dredge was as hard and nasty a job as there is. Everything was cold, wet, rusty, or oily. Mr. Ryan was so cheap he wouldn't buy rags; instead, he insisted we take the soiled rags home so our wives could wash them. Claudia would have none of that, so I bought rags from the marine store at the breakwater and charged them to my boss. This, another bone of contention, didn't improve our already shaky relationship.

One evening when the dredge sucked up a dead seal, the pump's vacuum came to a standstill. The massive cover plate had to be removed and the seal dismembered. The critter's decomposing body swelled with the heat of the engine room, and it appeared we would have to perform some serious surgery on the hairy corpse to free it. The stench was as bad as anything I have ever experienced – even worse than Mel on a hot day. (If that is possible.)

Mr. Ryan, investigating the shut-down, found Virgil, the engineer, and me covered with blood and rancid blubber. He took over the work himself and his suit was soon unrecognizable. Virgil interrupted him with, "Boss, haive you ever haid so much fun?"

With this, Mr. Ryan threw down his tools and left.

As mate, the scow was my responsibility. God how I hated the beast! A trip to the fuel dock was an experience few seamen have ever enjoyed.

This assemblage of boxes was almost as wide as it was long. The old Chrysler powered a large, three-bladed, cast-iron propeller with one blade missing. Because of this, the remaining two blades thrashed wildly at the water. During a turn, the prop's uneven wake would rip the large wheel right out of my hands. When I tried hanging on with my body weight, I usually ended up on the rusty steel deck while the scow headed for occupied waters.

Even when it was on a straight course through the center of the channel, the giant piece of crap would exercise her desire to go sideways at any time and in either direction. Any foolhardy attempt to straighten her up would put her into a side-slip, which occasionally ended in a collision with a yacht. The yacht and Mr. Ryan's insurance company always lost.

The only alternative was to turn her in the same direction in which she had started to rotate, and then do my best to straighten her once a full-circle had been executed – a "Crazy Ivan" in sub terms.

This maneuver would stop anyone who was observing it. The curious would stare. "Why did that nutty dredgerman suddenly pull a broady in the middle of the channel?"

Our round-the-clock operation required two shifts of twelve on, twelve off, with Saturdays included. I hated every minute of it but couldn't afford to give up the healthy paycheck. The city fathers then decided we were making too much noise at night, and they required the company to either re-power with electricity or lay off the evening crew. I got my walking papers and, though I missed the money, I was relieved.

The same city fathers then decided Phillip A. Ryan was getting rich, and too quick.

They bought their own dredge — the brand new *La Renna*. I have no idea how much she cost, but it was a lot. She was as cute as could be, even sported a galley and coffee mess in the leverman's cab. Unfortunately, she did not have enough power to pump the sand far enough to comply with the city's requirements. The fathers solved this problem by changing the specifications, reducing the length of the discharge line. The pipe's new end was very close to Stearns Wharf, almost where the sand had begun its journey in the first place.

As the city's dredging efforts fell behind, the sand mound grew. The grains of sand became polished from its many trips through the dredge and the pipe. Ten years later the sand bar was so high and the channel so shallow that some boats were required to anchor east of Stearns Wharf. In fact, no actual channel into the harbor existed.

In 1969 the city awarded a contract to reconstruct the entire harbor and it was decided that money could be saved if the city did its own dredging. The little *La Renna* was finally put down when she encountered a layer of large cobblestones, remnants of a glacier. She was then sold and towed away.

And yet another dredging firm was hired to resume polishing the sand. A task which still continues today.

For some time, I would occasionally receive a telephone call from the Ryan Construction Company requesting my welding services. Mr. Ryan would outline my task; then, out of earshot, he would tell his foreman to fire me when the welding was completed. I did the welding, but no love existed between the two of us.

Years later I ran into him at a restaurant in Santa Maria and we had lunch together. I felt somewhat sorry for him. His personality had not improved. Phillip A. Ryan was, and is, a hard man.

THE SKUNK WORKS, THE *SEAL*, AND THE *BEETLE*

My termination from the dredging business was not a heartbreaker, but it did present an immediate problem — my making a living. Claudia and I built a locked, roofed, green workbench behind the row of shops at the breakwater, and we survived by doing all sorts of odd jobs on yachts and commercial fishing boats. This green structure quickly became known as the "Skunk Works."

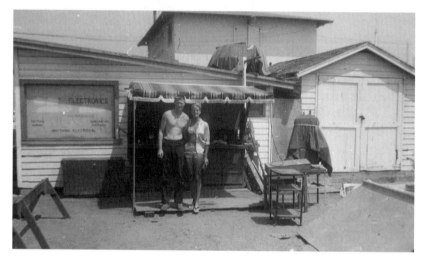

SKUNK WORKS, 1959

My bride was at my side most of the time, sanding, cleaning and polishing. I accepted every kind of task including the mechanical work which was my love.

We occasionally took on a job that was over our heads. On one such job, we were required to rout out the seams on a large teak deck and fill them with a new rubber compound, KemSeal, a thick, rubber goop that came in a one-gallon can and had to be mixed with a setting agent.

The mixing procedure would cause a most patient preacher to throw down his Bible and stomp on it. Most of the black slop ended up on Claudia or me and, after the steering wheel of our Chevy truck acquired a goopy texture, it remained that way. I couldn't come up with a good way to clean my hands, or anything else for that matter.

No one understood the product at the ship chandlers and, as an appeasement, they suggested using acetone to reduce the crap. Instead, the acetone reduced us to tears because the KemSeal was transformed into hundreds of black strands that clung to everything — spider webs from hell. Very soon, everything we owned smelled like KemSeal

― a pungent substance to say the least.

Refusing to be beat down, I fell back on my mechanical abilities. I modified an aluminum pressure cooker which allowed us to pump the KemSeal into the opened deck seams, but when I put pressure on my aluminum apparatus it exploded. KemSeal was everywhere ― on us, on the new docks, on the adjacent yachts, and on the skippers of same.

Several days passed before the gooey black substance finally made its way into the deck seams and we made any money. In the meantime my cleanup girl, who ended up looking like Little Black Sambo's wife, went through five gallons of acetone.

I started re-powering the older local fishing boats by replacing their turn-of-the-century one- and two-cylinder gas engines with modern diesels. I also devised a quick and very accurate method of mounting the modern mills on steel beds instead of the old timbers. I could build the beds and install the new engine in three days; that is if the controls didn't need to be rehashed. If the controls <u>did</u> need to be rebuilt, I could still have the boat underway in one week.

The *Seal* was one such boat. A very old fantail, the *Seal* was owned by Richard Headley. Richard was the kind of person you couldn't refuse. He captured seals for marine parks and zoos with an old tub that was in need of repairs. "Soon, perhaps in six months," he said, "we'll overhaul her. Okay, Kirby? But for now we'll use her the way she is."

"What do you mean, 'we'?" I wondered.

"Yeah, you can be my oarsman. All you have to do is row the skiff. I'll handle the seals. Come on Kirb. I know you'll love it."

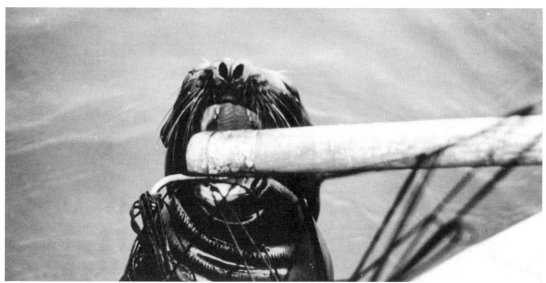

Richard Headley

SEAL BITING ON HOOK STICK

The fantail was about forty-five-feet long, and its bunks were forward in a small, independent house. On the first trip out her leaking decks poured water onto my sleeping bag, completely soaking it, and I spent one of the most miserable nights of my life.

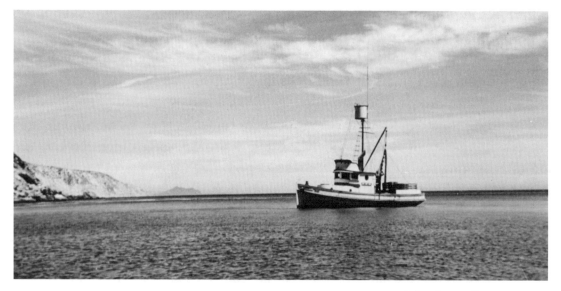

Richard Headley

SEAL ON ANCHOR

The *Seal* was powered by an old Frisco Standard fifteen-horse, two-lung, make-and-break gas engine. In 1905 it was probably the cat's behind; in 1959 it was sorely outdated. The crankcase belched unburned fuel, carbon monoxide, and oil, but this didn't seem to bother my salty skipper. "Dirty Dick the Seal Hunter" would open all the windows, breathe deeply, and proclaim our miserable existence as being heaven itself or very close to it.

Richard never got cold. I, on the other hand, never got warm while aboard. I spent my time looking for a place to get comfortable. Every spot on the *Seal* was wet, cold, oily and filled with an accumulation of terrible gases – or held a spike in the wrong place.

Starting the Frisco was a piece of work worth mentioning. A large, cast-iron flywheel rimmed with deep notches had to be turned by a steel bar inserted in one notch which was used as a lever to roll the two-ton vehicle through its compression cycle.

First, both igniters were unbolted, removed, and their contacts cleaned. They were then replaced, and a small shot of gasoline was squirted into two open petcocks to prime each cylinder. The make-and-break ignition flicker, a cam-operated spring and blade, was placed in the retarded position. This was to ensure the engine would start in the correct direction. If this important step was omitted, the starting bar would be flung backwards, cutting the *Seal* and its operator in half. Therefore, it seemed rather important to retard the ignition first.

112

The valves also had to be retarded. (I don't recall the reason for this, but I do remember that if this step was omitted, another equally unfortunate consequence could result.)

The flywheel was rotated with the switch in the off position. A slurping noise − resembling finishing off a milk shake with a straw − resulted. This meant the fuel was being sucked into the engine.

The next half-turn compressed the air and fuel within one of the large cylinders. Once the flywheel was at top dead center, the switch was turned on. A little more on the bar and the stack of oily castings would emit a muffled grunt. At this point the engine would either rotate or fart through its brass carburetor and start a gasoline fire.

The massive flywheel began its journey very slowly at first. The second compression stroke produced a smarter sound as the flywheel picked up speed. The operator then had to advance both the ignition and the valves. The grunts became muffled pops, and the engine was on its way to life − all fifteen horses worth.

The lubrication system worked on the total-loss method. A pump sent oil to various locations until it was eventually thrown off by the whirling crankshaft. Its last job was to saturate everything in the boat − the galley, the berths, my soggy sleeping bag, and the crew members who were stupid enough to be there in the first place.

Forward was direct drive and afforded the *Seal* a good six knots. To put the large diameter prop into reverse, a wheel in the flying bridge was turned counter-clockwise, and the chain in the engine room began to wind. This pulled the reverse lever back. At that point, the worn out gears started howling like a trapped wolf with a paw partially chewed off. The fantail would then begin to jump up and down as it backed into reverse.

This was not my first introduction to a Frisco Standard. In 1949 when I was about seventeen, I worked at the Palo Alto boat works for George Kuykendhall, another close friend. He owned a WWI captain's gig that was powered by a one-lung, five-horse Frisco. The twenty-three-foot black boat had a quarter hemisphere "whaleback" house on its bow with two portholes looking out at a forty-five-degree angle. It looked like a giant beetle, hence its name. I loved running this thing up, down, and around the muddy sloughs of the south bay.

Since the flywheel on the smaller Frisco was rolled over with a foot instead of a steel bar, failure to retard the ignition did not cut the operator in half; it merely broke his leg. The engine turned three-hundred revolutions per minute, producing a slow "pop pop" exhaust sound. The only problem was the engine shook like a small dog passing large peach pits. Each "pop" shook the *Beetle*'s bow to starboard and her stern to port. The steady vibration opened her seams, and the flywheel then threw oil bilge water from her engine box. This was no big deal; we got used to pumping her all the time.

Youth has it good points and its drawbacks. In those days I was pure. I loved girls; what I mean is I <u>really</u> liked them. And because my lady friends were as pure as me, my gonads had been complaining for some time. One day when I was washing down a boat bottom, George spotted two girls walking down the road. I don't know why they had taken this particular route because the road passed the city dump and terminated at the dilapidated boat works — neither of which could be referred to as a garden spot.

"Hey Red, look up the road," George said. "Offer to take them for a ride on the *Beetle*. Maybe they want to go swimming." George understood my predicament.

I couldn't believe my luck! Two available females, and they weren't wearing bathing suits! The heavy girl with big tits was covered with zits and her friend was very skinny. Oh well. Any port in a storm.

"Hi," I called out. "I'm Bob. How would you like to go for a boat ride, maybe go swimming or something like that."

Both started to giggle. "Okay," one replied.

They sat in the open cabin, watching my every move as I went through the starting routing. Soon the flywheel was spinning and the engine was pop-pop-popping. As predicted, the *Beetle* began its rhythmic shaking and leaking, and I cast off. Our odyssey began.

I had selected a slough about a quarter-of-a-mile away with a deep, clear basin at its end. I hoped to lose my virginity at this particular spot, and prospects were looking pretty good. As I rounded the bend and neared the swimming hole, the flywheel began throwing water out the open engine box. I began to pump at an easy pace, but as the overhead fan of oily water increased, I had to speed up my one-armed efforts. Soon I was pumping with both hands while I spun the wheel hard over. This turned the little *Beetle* in her own length, and I headed her homeward.

"Why are you turning around?" the girl with the tits and zits asked. "I thought we were going swimming." (She appeared to be the smarter of the two; the skinny girl just sat there. She apparently hadn't noticed we were heading back.)

"We <u>are</u> going swimming," I told them. "That's the problem."

When the *Beetle* reached the boat works dock, my female crew jumped ship, leaving me with a leaking boat and an erection.

During the night the boat took on so much water that it settled in the mud. The following morning after pumping her out, we hauled her up on the ways and sold her. I never saw the *Beetle* again.

*   *   *   *

Richard Headley is a gourmet today; in 1959, he was not. We planned to spend one day reaching San Miguel Island, forty miles west of Santa Barbara. We would hunt the second day and spend the third on a return-trip home where warmth beckoned.

I expected to see Dick load a large box of groceries, but I didn't question him when he boarded carrying only a small, brown paper bag. How stupid could I have been? He had made this trip many times, and I figured he knew the ropes. He certainly looked the part. His Barnacle-Jim-Penn-style skipper's cap should have been my first clue.

Once we were at sea, I asked what was for lunch.

"Nothing," he told me. "I brought only three tuna sandwiches for each of us. We'll have one sandwich this evening."

It was a long and miserable day. In an attempt to escape the *Frisco's* foul belching, I tried sitting in the bow and I got drenched. I tried both the flying bridge and wheelhouse and was gassed in both locations. Cold, nauseous, and hungry, I attempted to sleep; then discovered my bag was once again soaked in cold, oily seawater. Six hours into our trip, the sea began to build. I pointed out to my captain that we would be unable to set our nets if it got any rougher.

"Don't worry, Kirb. If it gets too rough, we'll anchor out in the eastern harbor overnight. We might even row ashore and look the place over."

The seas were so high that, by the time we reached the anchorage, it was all we could do to make it safely over the bar. It was still early afternoon, and we had a lot of time to kill. Richard launched his flat-bottomed seal skiff, and we pushed away towards the breaker-lined beach.

As Richard rowed, he looked the part of a true skipper; blue turtleneck under a denim shirt, cap mashed squarely on his head, broad shoulders pulling smartly against the green sea. For sure, we were on our way to an adventure.

Any good seaman knows that, though beaching a skiff is a standard procedure, it is a procedure that must be executed with care. Long before reaching the breaker zone, the boat must be turned around with its bow into the oncoming waves. Then it is backed in. If the boat is caught by a large wave, the oarsman can maintain control by pulling hard forward and keeping his bow straight into the wave, thus avoiding an uncontrolled surf ride ending in a life-threatening broach. If broached, the skiff usually capsizes in this unfortunate situation, and the occupants are submerged and tossed about in the cold and sand-filled water.

As we neared the beach, our keel slid over large waves and we were lifted four or five feet before the water receded and settled us back down. The walls of water were growing in size. By now, I thought, my skipper should be turning us into the high swells. But maybe he knew something I didn't...

Then a very mature wave picked us up, and we were quickly skimming down its face at a high rate of speed; two surfers on a long board that was out of control.

The little boat began its predictable broach and, as it turned sideways, I slid off my seat and got under, holding on for all I was worth. The last view I had of my captain, Dick was sitting smartly where he had been, oars in hand, hat on head, as he turned upside-down within the cold, green froth.

I sensed an endless, fierce passage of time. My cheeks filled with sand and my head was violently shaken; I felt as if I was being flushed down a gigantic toilet. Then, except for a soft hissing sound as the water receded, all noise ceased. I was submerged, trapped under the rear seat and holding my breath. The skiff, filled with water, was sealed to the sand by its gunnels. Then the boat began to rise. As Richard pushed it off himself, I was also freed. Then we both pushed. We were now standing at the side of the boat, two men very lucky to be alive.

Suddenly, an even larger wave broke over us, washing us and the boat against the rocks. I was bruised; even worse, the chine and one side of the boat were badly smashed and one of the oars had broken in two, rendering it useless.

Pulling the skiff to higher ground, Dick and I assessed our situation. The *Seal* was anchored out, probably too far for us to make it swimming. We possessed one smashed skiff, one oar, and we were wet and very cold. Richard's handgun, a stupid idea to begin with, was full of sand and getting rusty. We were both pissed off, but I'm sure I was angrier than my salty captain.

Grabbing a rock, I pounded the broken wood roughly into shape. Then I began carving a sculling notch into the transom. "No Kirby!" Richard yelled. "Not my beautiful stern!"

"Tough shit, Richard." I told him. "This is how it is. I want to get back to the *Seal* and eventually home to something warm; maybe even something to eat besides tuna fish and bread. Give me a hand, you asshole."

By the grace of God, we made it back through the breakers. Sitting on one side to keep the damage above water, I sculled like a possessed demon until we reached the comforting decks of the old fishing boat. Little or no dialogue transpired between us on our way back to Santa Barbara.

My salty captain hates me for bringing up this episode, a tale I refer to as "Dirty Dick The Seal Hunter." I always enjoy recalling the story at fancy parties where he is revered as a god. His new friends don't have a clue as to the not-so-funny joke.

Richard and I eventually rebuilt the *Seal*, and I worked as his oarsman for several more trips. We enjoyed dry sleeping bags, clean air, healthy hot meals, and even managed to capture some of the little critters.

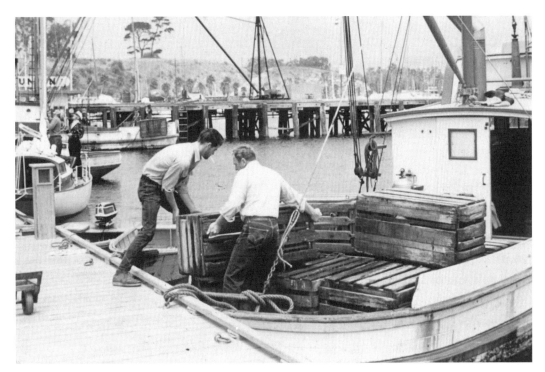

RICHARD UNLOADING SEALS

We loved the seals and did our best not to harm them. Most of those that end up on the beach had died of a prevalent venereal disease similar to the human variety. To assure ourselves of having caught a healthy, young female, Richard had to pull her rear flippers over the stern of the skiff and run his fingers into the vagina to inspect it. Let me tell you, sticking your finger into a seal's pussy gets the seal's attention real fast. This is one reason the skiff's gunwales were protected by stainless steel.

A large bull got tangled up in our net once, and it took us a good half hour to free him. By then he was enraged and did his best to climb into the skiff with us. Richard asked what I thought we should do if he were to succeed.

"Dick," I told him, "I'm going to get into the seal crate and close the door. What are you going to do?"

Richard continued hunting seals for several more years. Eventually he sold his sealing license and leased the fantail.

The new owner of the *Seal* was out with a fish and game biologist. The two got into trouble and had to be towed in by a coast guard cutter. The cutter's skipper went too fast, and the *Seal* broached, rolled, and was pulled under. The fisherman was saved, but the biologist did not return to his office.

The biologist and the *Seal* were never found, and the coast guard skipper was reprimanded and transferred from his command in warm Santa Barbara to a position tending a lighthouse in Barrow, Alaska. Perhaps this is where he belonged in the first place.

THE GREAT SEA SCOUT CAPER

The hull of our thirty-foot ketch cleanly parted the brown waters of San Francisco's south bay on its way through the many muddy channels. Sails full, the vessel answered smartly as our mate pushed the tiller away and called out, "Coming about!"

All hands set down their beer cans and tended to the many lines that had to be hauled in, readjusted, and secured. As our sails refilled, my fellow sea scouts and I raised our cans to our eager lips, then broke into yet another filthy song.

> "'Open the door and lay on the floor,' cried Barnacle Bill the Sailor.
> 'Open the door and lay on the floor,' cried Barnacle Bill the Sailor.
> 'What if my parents should find out?' What if my parents should find out?
> 'What if my parents should find out?' cried the fair young maiden.
> 'To hell with your pa, forget your ma,' cried Barnacle Bill the Sailor.
> 'To hell with your pa, forget your ma,' cried Barnacle Bill the Sa-ai-lor."

I spent three years in the sea scouts during high school, 1947-1950. My mother was delighted, for she thought I was singing songs of loyalty and goodness while learning to tie knots. She never suspected that my deranged shipmates and I had joined in order to get drunk and learn the words to every dirty song known to man.

An enlistment bonus was our skipper's well-rounded young wife. When she went swimming in her bra and panties, the fabric became transparent. Then she would prance around the ship's decks. Several of my shipmates were invited to entertain her while our skipper was at work but, darn, not me. What a great way to earn a merit badge!

It was just as well she didn't take to me because my mates ended up with a dose of the clap. One of the survivors of this jolly crew was my friend, Wayne "Dynamite" Smithson. Dynamite earned his handle when the two of us decided the best way to remove the booty of brass fittings that adorned the many wrecks of the south bay waters was to blow them off with dynamite.

On our way to Cupertino, then a farming village near San Jose, we stopped my 1937 Dodge to give a Mexican orchard worker a lift. "Amigo," I said, "want to earn a dollar for doing nothing?"

I brought him with me into the hardware store. "Sir," I said, addressing the clerk, "I need a case of forty percent, two dozen caps, and fifteen feet of fuse. My helper and I have to blast some stumps in my dad's orchard."

The clerk didn't doubt me for a minute, for I had picked up the correct terminology from my uncle who worked in a gold mine during the war. I further enhanced my credibility (and survivability) by putting the case of powder in the trunk and the caps in the glove box.

While I played a very convincing powder monkey, I was still a virgin when it came to dynamite and girls. I had yet to light my first fuse or dip my wick. On the way home we came upon two girls who were hitchhiking — strictly a no-no in those days. Wayne spoke up with, "Hi. How would you like to go swimming?"

Giggle giggle and an "Okay." How stupid can you get.

When we reached the edge of the lake, Wayne commanded them to take off their clothes. "Here?" one asked. "In the car?"

"Sure," Wayne told her. "If you don't, I'll set off this stick of dynamite and blow them off."

The girls ran like hell, I remained a virgin, Wayne acquired his nickname, "Dynamite," and I never forgave him.

Out in a muddy slough that afternoon we had only partial success blowing the brass fittings off an old landing craft. Just for the fun of it, our attacks became more flamboyant. We began by blowing up the catwalks to the many duck blinds. A properly secured, double-shaped charge, above and below, sent the wood spinning spectacularly. Then we escalated into blowing up empty hunting shacks — most of them were loosely constructed with scrap wood and grass. Our efforts put previous Fourth of July thrills to shame.

A good-sized charge ended up in one of the muddy ponds that the stingray population of the bay called home. We were amazed how wildly a stingray flapped when his equilibrium was destroyed.

By the end of the day, only twenty sticks of dynamite remained. That night Wayne told his parents how we had spent the day and, for some reason, they became very upset. My mother was alerted, a fleet of cops arrived, the explosives in the trunk of my Dodge were confiscated, and I received a stern warning.

Looking back, I can't decide whether my day spent with Wayne or the day Jerry Todd put me down was the best day of my life. I guess the explosives win out. If I had lost my virginity and enjoyed a can of beer, I would have probably died in ecstasy.

* * * *

I was delighted when I discovered Santa Barbara had a sea scout troop and an ex-navy power boat. I expected to find these young sea scouts as well-versed in dirty lyrics as I had been. To my dismay, I discovered just the opposite. Raised on milk toast and protected from men like me, they knew little of the sea, the running of a boat, or life in general. I felt sorry for them.

Even sorrier was their worn out WWII captain's gig. This derelict was one of many navy vessels that had been loaned to sea scouts throughout the country after WWII. Unlike our San Francisco Bay troop, the Santa Barbara scouts did no maintenance. When it came to mechanics, they were as ignorant as their skipper must have been. Instead of actually going to sea and getting drunk, their time was spent sailing dinghies and answering with an "Aye aye, sir."

I was saddened by the condition of their captain's gig, especially when I learned that a desirable, 6-71 GMC diesel engine was rusting away in her oily engine room. One morning the old vessel surrendered to neglect as she submerged in the harbor's cool waters. Traces of oil remained as evidence of her once-proud self.

Since no one actually owned the boat, no one had given a thought to her ultimate end. Who pays for its removal? I wondered. Who owns its parts? What if it was a hazard to navigation? My concerns were ignored. Still, as a good patriotic American, I felt it was my duty to do something about the situation. Another disaster waiting to happen was the sunken gig's two domed houses lying only seven feet under the surface of the water. They could be snagged by a passing yacht or fishing boat. Or the wreck could be sucked into the cutter of the city's new dredge. That wonderful 6-71 engine would then go to waste.

I, of course, had a personal interest in the gig. I had recently won a contract to design and build a new harbor patrol boat, and I could use the brass hardware that was now under water.

So I turned to my friend, Joe Greco, a thin, six-foot-three Sicilian known as "The Lonesome Polecat." Joe's WWII landing craft, the *El Greco* was powered by two 6-71s and, over a cup of coffee, I convinced him he could use a spare engine. "Come on," I urged, "let's steal it. Who will know the difference? We'll be doing everyone a service."

Joe had a reputation for helping out whenever someone needed a boat for a dirty job but, since I last encountered him (provoked by a night in jail due to an unfortunate understanding) Joe had acquired a new attitude. "No way," he insisted. "We have to go to the scout council and plead our case."

Joe's recent troubles began when he decided not to push his luck by continuing to drive the 1946 Plymouth Business Coupe he had been driving (unlicensed), one mile and back, to the breakwater every day for seven years. Using the large crane on the end of Stearns Wharf, he loaded his car onto the bow of his *El Greco* and, in order to keep it from rolling off, he tied the car down. Then he ran about a mile out to Camby's Reef, cut the lines, and dumped the car in the briny. He assumed that was the end of his problem.

Unknown to my lanky friend, a girl was missing in Santa Barbara and suspicion spread that she might be in the trunk of Joe's Plymouth. After a night in jail, Joe was convinced the authorities were serious. The sunken car would have to be inspected.

Soon an armada of boats were dragging the reef — fathometers were still new and not very accurate — and a host of SCUBA divers were involved. By the end of the day, it was determined that Mr. Greco had played no part in the girl's disappearance, but two problems remained. One, the car had not been registered. Two, who was going to pay for the search? Joe simply waited it out and, eventually, the problems went away. (The incident did leave its wounds, however. Several years later the wife of the now-famous "Polecat" filed for divorce.)

Returning to my original story; Joe and I drove to the scout office where the head of the council told us, "Hell yes. Get the thing out of the channel...but there is a glitch...the navy still owns it...if it should turn up 'missing'...that's how it is."

That evening we loaded the *El Greco* with the diving gear I had built in partnership with Bob Benton, one of the famous Benton brothers. When we reached the site of the wreck, we were amazed to find a sea scout boat from Ventura anchored over it. We tied alongside Charlie Isbell's derrick barge and watched as young scuba divers brought up treasures, mainly engine parts. Joe was very upset, but the dive boat eventually departed, no doubt assuming that "tomorrow will be another day." A big surprise was in store for them.

As day turned to night, we anchored over the wreck. Because I was experienced, diving with no visibility, I felt quite at home. All I had to do was run one hogging line under the gig's bow and another under its stern. We tied them off to cleats on the *El Greco* and Joe hit the throttles. The gig pulled free of the sandy bottom and was on its way to another temporary home, on the bottom alongside the derrick barge. The two lines were loosely tied to cleats, handy for rigging.

Around ten the following morning, the Ventura Sea Scout boat returned, and a young diver went over its side. we watched as his bubbles wandered; then a very dismayed argonaut surfaced.

"What the hell do you mean, its not there?" Their leader exclaimed. "It has to be! Get out of the water, I'll take a look."

The young scout was correct, of course, and we soon saw only the wake of the boat from Ventura as it slipped out of the harbor and headed south.

Securing the hogging lines to the load block of the crane, I pulled back on the crane's lever and the wreck rose to the surface. Once she had drained, I set her on deck. The Lonesome Polecat got the engine and I ended up with all the brass fittings, the rudder, shaft, strut bearing, prop, and packing gland.

The patrol boat that I built with the salvaged parts lasted twenty years, a testimony to Fellows and Stewart, the shipwrights who had built the salvaged gig during the war. If the city fathers had known the parts were over twenty years old when I installed them, they would have been very upset. Tee hee.

Joe and I shared many adventures before he contracted cancer in the late eighties, and the grim reaper took him away. The Santa Barbara Sea Scouts continued to sail their dinghies, and I imagine they never did learn anything about nuts, bolts, grease, wine, women, song, and debauchery.

What a tragedy. A young mind is a terrible thing to waste.

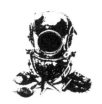

THE WRETCHED *REX*

Fat ladies here,
Some falling there.
the stem of the *Rex*
Is beyond repair.
I hold on tight
It's a wonder we float
I curse the day
I skippered this boat.

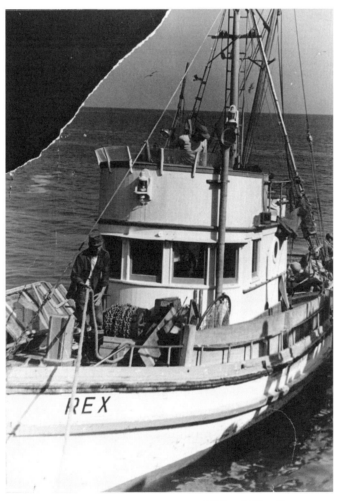

Richard Headley

THE *REX*

123

Before offshore oil was developed in Santa Barbara, fishing was the largest local offshore industry. The Castagnola family, George, Mario, and their cousins, owned several boats. As the fish population dwindled, George and Mario, now the successful owners of George V. Castagnola Sea Foods and proud of their background as fishermen, kept just one boat, George V.'s pride and joy, the fifty-five-foot long *Rex*.

The boom days of offshore oil rewarded any boat that would float, and George V. turned his wooden dragger into a work boat, supplying Platform Hilda off Summerland, the first oil production jacket.

Wooden boats do not fair well around steel structures. Soon the rails of the *Rex* were missing; next to go was her uppermost planking. The old craft needed a serious facelift; a facelift requiring vast amounts of lumber, paint, and loving care or she would sink on her next voyage.

George V. and Dick Headley, Mario's stepson, came over to the shop where I built the harbormaster's boat, and the fish buyers convinced me to assume the task of rebuilding the once-proud *Rex*. I was probably foolish to accept the one-year contract without first inspecting the vessel.

Before I could start on her rusty, forlorn engine room, I had to replace rails that had been torn away and replace planks and decks with beautiful new timbers. These jobs took six weeks.

God's earth holds countless engines of all colors and descriptions, but only one truly wonderful model — the Caterpillar D-13000 — is fine enough to take home and put in your living room. That is, if your living room is large enough to hold it.

This cast-iron beast was covered with rust, peeling paint, and oil, but she ran like new, puffing out her slow and steady bursts of brute power. To start the engine, you pulled back the diesel's compression release and then started a two-cylinder, gasoline pony engine with a hand crank. You then had to engage the starting gear and clutch. The engine began to rotate and warm up. As you opened the throttle, small gray puffs of exhaust burst from her stack accompanied by the burps and belches of uneven power strokes. Soon the yellow mass became a living thing, roaring with all one-hundred ponies in a row, a delight for any sailor.

We think of horsepower today in terms of automobile horses — many animals jumping up and down, here and there. The old Cat, however, had a team of Clydesdales — hard-working draft horses with slow-moving, powerful legs and enormous feet. When the Cat began to rotate the thirty-eight-inch-diameter prop, a torrent of water erupted from under the fantail. The *Rex* was then underway in a grand manner that only a seaman could appreciate.

This job completed, I still had to rebuild the *Rex's* steering and reverse gear. Some "brilliant" engineer had specified that the huge steering wheel required nine revolutions from one hard stop to the other. The wheel was also difficult to turn and, before we were free of the harbor, my shoulders would feel as though they were falling off. After I rebuilt the entire system, it required five turns and the wheel spun with ease.

The hydraulic reversing gear was a bigger problem. It had been given to George V. by the Western Gear Company in 1958, when hydraulic marine gearboxes were innovations. The original plan was for him to test it in the dragger, an almost fatal mistake. No skipper could subdue this monster. It took twelve seconds for the transmission to respond to the reversing lever, and trying to think ahead twelve seconds in a large battering ram like the *Rex* was like playing Russian roulette with half the chambers loaded.

Because of the faulty valving inside the reversing gearbox, mishap after mishap resulted. Once in a while the thing would go into forward gear all by itself. This occurred so rarely that, assuming the problem had gone away, the owners let down their guards.

I had forgotten about this hazard myself until one day when, surrounded by commercial vessels just off Stearns Wharf, I had the engine pulled back to an idle as I prepared anchoring tackle on the aft deck. I heard the engine take a load, then the prop began to churn, and suddenly we were making three knots of headway. I ran to the wheelhouse, making it just in time to avoid a disaster.

George V. soon had me skippering the old boat, doing all sorts of tasks. One operation involved towing a large barge to Platform Hilda to deliver drilling pipe and mud. The wood barged leaked like mad. Its owner would not put a cent into maintaining it, so I had to keep her pumped all day and night.

One day George V. called and said, "Red, a team of photographers wants to do a beer commercial off East Beach. I think it's Lucky Lager Beer. Have the *Rex* and the barge alongside the wharf at seven."

This was my first encounter with movie people, and I had no idea their system was so complex. We had to load cameras, lights, extension cords, reflectors, generators, and many other boxes of essential equipment, all attended to by a large crew of young men and women wearing shorts. A catering service within a small trailer was also lifted aboard.

We pulled away from Stearns Wharf with the barge tied alongside the *Rex*; the barge was completely covered with equipment and personnel.

Everyone was complaining about the clatter of the engine-powered bilge pump, a necessity for keeping the barge afloat. I assured them I could shut it down for a couple of hours, but I didn't bother to explain the barge would take on several tons of water and become unstable in the meantime.

They were after footage of a bikini-clad water skier passing by and throwing a high spray. Just as she passed a beer was opened and poured into a glass, accompanied by the jingle, "*It's lucky when you live in America...it's Lucky Lager Beer.*"

My wife and friend Tory with his new wife had a perfect view from the flying bridge of the *Rex*. The ski boat would fly by, beer would flow, and the actors would then toss it over the side! "Hey there," we yelled, "don't chuck it overboard. Give it to us!"

It was a long day. Take after take, beer after beer — all of which ended up in our bellies. Soon quite drunk, I was forced to take a nap.

"Hey Kirby, they want to go in." Tory was standing over me. I got to my feet and headed for the engine room, still groggy. After I had the mill started, a task taking much longer than it should, I pulled up the anchor. Once in gear, the huge horse in that magnificent old Cat pushed the *Rex* and the barge, now partially filled with water, at a good speed. With the wind blowing in my hair, I felt like Gregory Peck — very nautical even if I wasn't wearing a skipper's cap.

As we approached the pier I cut back the throttle, but my judgement was impaired. We were much closer than I had realized. I threw the engine into reverse and, after an agonizing wait, it took the load and great mounds of water boiled up from beneath the *Rex*. Filled with water, the barge was now extremely heavy, and it would have been difficult to stop her even if I hadn't been full of Lucky Lager Beer.

We slammed into the wharf with the force of an earthquake.

The result was an unbelievable mess — I had overturned the drinks and rearranged the plates of food in two restaurants on the pier, people were laying all over the deck of the barge, and the equipment was scattered everywhere. The movie crew's prized generator had taken a swim and it was not retrieved for several hours. Everyone seemed to be upset.

Still handicapped but using extreme caution, I took the *Rex* and the barge back into the harbor. George Castagnola was never again called upon to film a commercial, I never again drank while operating the boat, and Tory never again sailed with me. Perhaps a lesson was learned, but I doubt it.

For years, "Maria Macaroni," had been the flamboyant hostess of Santa Barbara's annual "Battle of the Flowers," a parade of fishing boats honoring the sea. Maria was perhaps seventy, slightly plump, and she wore a fluffy short full skirt and revealing peasant top from which her large bosom was on the verge of escaping. You knew, by her set jaw and piercing eyes, Maria was sure of herself and the task she had to accomplish. She only had time for hard work; games and foolishness were not tolerated. She strutted down the navy pier, giving orders and calling out blessings to the fishermen, her full skirt and long, silver hair blowing in the breeze.

Because the Battle of the Flowers was a thanksgiving for God's creatures, the fishing boats were to be ornamented with palm fronds, flowers, and wreaths. The owner of the

Rex, a firm believer in the event's significance, overruled my wishes and ordered me to take on the task, like it or not. Maria and her boarding party swept onto the old dragger armed with a truckload of hammers, palm fronds, and sixteen-penny nails.

I attempted to stop her crew from nailing the fronds to the wheelhouse because this would leave holes in the *Rex's* wonderful woodwork, but I was no match for this full-bodied, female leader. She and her team continued to pound, contaminating the *Rex* with rusty nails. "These are beautiful," she insisted. "Many flowers, all blessed by the Father. You will see. He will bless you as well. Your life will change for the better."

The ebullient Maria was dashing around in every direction, bouncing off objects. She jumped onto the aging *Monterey* owned by an old Greek fisherman and urged him to join the festivities. He was going to resist until he spotted her breasts, and then he invited her to tour his fo'c'sle. Once he got her there, he pulled down her blouse and her splendid bosom was exposed. By the time she made it back up the ladder, screaming like a calliope, his hands were up her dress and his trousers were unfastened.

Back aboard the *Rex,* Maria seemed strangely subdued, and she was smiling a soft, Mona Lisa smile. Our guess was she had realized she still had "it," and someone wanted "it." Not bad for a woman her age. There was a new sparkle in her eyes and her jaw, harshly set a little earlier, had relaxed. We were happy for her.

Then I got the bad news. The *Rex* would be leading the parade, her fine lines hidden behind a forest of thick, tropical foliage. What a sad way to display a working craft.

A priest stood on the navy pier, blessed all, and sprinkled us with holy water. Untying our lines, we headed out the channel with Maria standing on the bow, waving a wreath of bright flowers and shouting blessings. The parade, a long armada of fishing craft, followed dutifully in the wake of the *Rex.*

When we reached Summerland, our turn-around point, many spectators were lined up along the shore, sharing in the splendor. It is surprising how close one must get before realizing that sunbathers are not wearing clothing. We were sailing off the beach that has been recognized as a nude beach for over half a century. (Actually, I knew exactly what I was doing!)

Two people swam out to greet us, and when Maria discovered they were nude she acted as if she'd seen the devil himself. "Turn around!" she insisted. "Take me back!" Following her orders, I opened the throttle and we were soon making ten knots over and through the water, some of which came over the bow rail soaking Maria's silver hair and flowing dress which had now become a see-through model. "Slow down!" she yelled. "Do you think this is a race?!"

It was for me! I needed the companionship of normal people plus a drink.

Once in the harbor Maria, seeking other company, abandoned ship.

She succeeded in finding it, for that evening her fluffy white skirt was hanging over the life vests in the Greek fisherman's fo'c'sle. The Battle of the Flowers would never be the same.

* * * *

"Once a year the *Rex* takes all my fish-processing workers to the islands for a day of fishing," George V. told me. "Be here at six. Don't bother with food for the others, only for yourself." George V. was my boss and he was not a man to whom you said no.

Claudia and I had just purchased a brand new trailer with all the amenities, and we had moved into a fine new trailer park. There we were introduced to fellow occupants Woody Treen and his wife, Meribeth. Woody owned Treen's Commercial Diving Service, and I would start working part-time for him as soon as I returned from the fishing trip to the islands which would complete my year of obligation to George V.

When I asked Woody to accompany me on the fishing trip, he was delighted. "Bring your scuba gear," I told him. "We might be able to round up some abs or a bug."

Because the *Rex* had been hauling supplies to the oil patch, her decks had been protected by large planks. The surface of the deck was too uneven for my passengers, so I stacked the planks on each side for seating. I nailed the planks together securely, so they would not break apart on the trip. The twenty guests who showed up included a couple of very heavy ladies and one very thin male fish cutter. Some guests had brought enough fishing gear to outfit all the others.

After I had filled every nook and cranny of the wheelhouse with cardboard boxes containing food, access to the engine room was tight while access to the downstairs controls was almost impossible. We were further hindered by the two sets of scuba gear which I had squeezed into the flying bridge where Woody and I were situated. "Oh well," I thought. "I can live with this for one day."

If ever there was a boat that rolled it was the *Rex*. Her bilges were very round and her wheelhouse and bridge were heavily constructed − the old dragger would even roll at the dock. At sea, the only way to ride her out was to brace yourself against the side of the flying bridge with one foot on the wheel.

Three hours later we pulled in close to a wash rock south of Pelican Harbor. All lines went over the side and were soon tangled together. After a couple hours fishing, the guests began working together and, after another hour, we had a couple sacks of fish.

I decided to run the bow of the *Rex* closer to a huge rock to see if we could do better. There was no wind, and the smooth sea gave us a gently roll. Everything was great except my grand old engine was idling far too fast.

I headed down the ladder to the engine room to cut it back, leaving Woody at the controls. I had to squeeze through a narrow path between the large hindquarters of the ladies and the contents of the now-open boxes. As I parted the blubber, I heard the engine beginning to huff black smoky exhaust and take its load. We were underway and on a collision course with the rock, for I had forgotten to warn Woody about the treacherous Western Gear.

I dashed over the passengers like a monkey, desperate to reach the reverse lever in time. Reaching it, I pulled the handle aft, but there was no response. Then, after a very long five seconds, we struck the rock head on.

During a severe accident, everything seems to take place in slow motion. First there was a grinding of wood and rock, then the volume increased as we slowly climbed the jagged face of the rock. The screams from within our bilges sounded as if someone was dying and seemed to go on forever. By the time we had crawled to the top of the rock, the fishing boat had rolled over and was now at a forty-five-degree angle, and the accumulation of boxes, gear, and people within the wheelhouse had been further rearranged. Worse, far worse, all the planks had come loose on the afterdeck and were scattered between the fishermen and their tackle.

The reverse gear finally answered my command. As we slowly retreated back down the jagged rock and into the calm seas, the noise emanating from our torn keel was horrendous.

It is impossible to accurately express the thoughts that run through a skipper's head during a catastrophe like this. My passengers lives were in jeopardy, as was the life of the *Rex.* My own life was at risk as well; for even if we made it home, George V.'s Italian code might demand my feet to be cast in cement and my white body to be fed to the crabs on Camby's Reef.

Still in slow motion, I observed the destruction. Absolutely nothing was in order. People, sprawled everywhere, were laying on top of, and tangled within, broken fishing rods, fishing line, bait, tackle, and wooden planks. The screams of the women were louder than those of the bilges, and the men were in a daze. As rapidly as possible, I regained the controls and put her into forward before she could back down towards deep water. After another agonizingly long five seconds, she responded. I headed her straight for a sandy beach, hoping I could run her up on the sand and save everyone before she sank.

Then, on the way in, I noticed we had not settled in the water. Perhaps we would not sink after all. I stopped her in shallow water, turning her so as to lay sideways to the beach in case the Western Gear decided to replay its unpredictable game. I inspected the bilges and discovered they were dry. We would not sink. George V. would not be forced to kill me; instead, he would probably take everything I owned as repayment for the damage.

We anchored in Pelican Bay, an inlet protected by high rock cliffs on three sides. After patching the passengers back together (amazingly, no one was hurt), and restacking the planks, Woody and I donned our scuba gear for a close look at the damage.

Woody was a junk collector, and the scuba regulator he brought for me must have been purchased at a swap meet in Mexico. It contained a rectangular diaphragm; one of the first single-hose regulators manufactured. As soon as I hit the water, the damn thing flooded.

Woody returned to the surface after inspecting the damage. "Come on Kirby," he said, "take a look."

"How do I do that?" I asked. "Hold my breath?" Eventually purging the hose, I got enough air to look at the keel. Wood, eighteen-inches deep from the turn of the stem to the straight-run keel, was missing. The entire outer stem was gone. Eight feet of wood and steel was impaled on the rock for a future archaeologist to discover. I could imagine his reaction, "Okay, but where is the rest of the wreck?"

We determined the *Rex* was seaworthy enough to make it back to Santa Barbara, and our shaken guests fished for another couple of hours. George V. was standing on the dock when we returned, and he was eager for a report.

Unbeknownst to George V., the following day Woody and I constructed a temporary cement stem, fitted underwater.

Several months later, the day before the *Rex* was scheduled to leave for San Pedro and its annual haul-out, Sam Farris accidentally backed into it with his thirty-five-foot work boat. Neither vessel was damaged, but many onlookers who had witnessed the harmless collision reported it to George V. A month later the *Rex* returned, sporting a new stem, and Sam was presented with a bill for $5000. This was in 1959 when a brand new Chevy cost only $2000, so Farris rolled up the bill and did his best to shove it up George V.'s rectum.

The cat was now out of the bag. When my ex-boss heard the real story, he hired a cement truck and tried to fit me for a permanent pair of weighted shoes.

Steel boats soon filled the Santa Barbara Harbor, replacing all the old wooden boats that had done their best to supply the oil patch. The *Rex* was sold to fishermen who put it back to work as a dragger. They installed a faulty, propane stove valve, allowing the heavy gas to accumulate in her hull. The following morning, a mile from where the original stem remains on the island, someone lit a match and the craft blew up, killing the crew and sending the wonderful old dragger to Davy Jones.

I understand the Western Gear Company ceased production of its reverse gears.

George V. never stopped looking for me, though I imagine he tried until the day he died.

WOODY TREEN AND HIS BLUE-GREEN MACHINES

Come on, Bob,
Build me a hat
If you do it this week,
You can dive with that.
If you do not,
You're in the Mark V
You will then be lucky
To get out alive.

Now that the *Rex* was out of my life, I could start diving for Woody. However, on the first day of my employment, Woody had a very serious automobile accident and suffered massive head injuries. He couldn't dive for a year, and he couldn't work in the shop for six months. When he returned, his recently fractured skull would cause him to see things from a different point of view. Now a bit paranoid, Woody was a different man than he had been before the accident. Nevertheless, the small, handsome man continued to be a good salesman, and he began to gather in work.

Meribeth, his wife, called. "Woody just got a call from Richfield Oil. They want an inspection of the causeway to Rincon Island. I'll have him come over and talk to you."

Woody arrived. "Okay, here's the rundown. My tender, Willie, has the gear loaded in my pickup. All we have to do is meet the *Aquarius*, the Richfield VIP boat, at the navy pier at seven, load the gear, and be on our way. The job should be easy. Don't bother to bring lunch, we'll be home by noon."

"What gear?" I wondered.

"You know," Woody answered. "The Mark V. It's in great shape and I have a good dress as well."

God, how I hated those terrible helmets. I had sworn never again to use one, and now I was anticipating spending a day in misery, trying to look out of a view port smaller than the distance my eyes are apart.

I did not suspect I had much more in store for me that day than just a dinky view port. For that matter, I would be leaving a blight on my diving career that would never go away.

"What size dress do you have?" was my next question.

"Don't worry, it's big enough to dance in. And the gear is in great shape because we just overhauled it."

At that time, I didn't realize his mind had blanked out during the one-year recovery period, and though he was remembering having worked on the gear just the other day, he had actually worked on it over a year earlier. Also, as I was soon to learn, a businessman Woody was; a mechanic he was not.

The Richfield boat was a beautiful yacht, a converted navy torpedo boat with two giant Hall Scott gas hogs beneath her decks. Her brass was polished, as was Verne Wadell, her skipper, who was wearing a khaki outfit, carefully pressed, with a small Richfield logo on the pocket. A cocky type, fast and small, he wouldn't give anyone the time of day unless they arrived in a Rolls, and he treated me as if I was a pile of doggy poo. By the end of that day, Verne would hate me. And, looking back, he would have good reason.

Once underway, I noticed we lacked a diving ladder, a necessity when using heavy gear — especially when the yacht's decks are five feet above the water — and I questioned Willie about this oversight.

"Don't worry, Kirby. Verne said he has a Jacob's ladder. He prefers it because steel ladders scrape up his boat." Willie was not a convincing liar. I knew he had simply forgotten this essential piece of gear.

At twenty knots, it was a half-hour run to the Rincon Island. When we arrived we met Russell Fox, Richfield's Santa Barbara area superintendent. Joe Greco and I had worked with "Foxy" before, and we got along great. Perhaps the day might not be too bad after all — if I could make it back on board the sparkling boat, that is, and I had serious doubts. (My stool, an inverted metal milk box, had scratched the smooth, gray deck and Verne, in a huff, had placed a rubber mat under the spot where I was being dressed in before returning to his wheelhouse to pout.)

The dress seemed rather small, and I soon discovered it was very old and had been Woody's personal dress. Woody was five-five; I was six feet. When they tried to pull the holes in the collar of the dress up over the breastplate studs, they would not reach. I had to stand to afford as much slack material as possible, and then the dress's crotch was pulled up and into my butt. Heaving, pulling, and swearing, they finally had the holes over the studs, but now each was so stretched that the elongated holes protruded from beneath the brales. Massive leaking was imminent.

Once the brale nuts were tightened, I couldn't sit, bend my knees, or bend at the waist. I felt as if I was sewn into stiff leather after being embalmed in preparation for my funeral.

I did my best to walk to the rail, but with lead weights on my boots and my fifty-pound weight belt, my steps were choppy and hesitant. Foxy gave me the rundown. "After you inspect all the piles from the bottom up, come back to the boat. I'll give you a swell indicator to secure to the center of the offshore pile."

"All the piles...." We didn't have enough hose to cover half of them. Willie put on my hat, I jumped off the boat, and two seconds later I encountered the bottom with the force of an anchor. Air was leaking out of every fitting, all the brale holes, and everywhere else. The dress was rotten. I tried to blow up but couldn't retain enough air in my dress to do so. I had no control over my buoyancy and was instantly flooded. A predictable beginning for what was becoming a very bad day.

I did my best to make my way to the row of pilings and begin my inspection. Since I couldn't bend my knees, my method of locomotion was to pull myself along on my belly with my fingers while wiggling my toes a little. Very little.

I reported that the condition of the first pile at the sand line was excellent. Then I somehow managed to stand erect and make a second inspection at eye level. Again, when I attempted to blow up in order to view the pile above, I couldn't do it. I tried to do my job, crawling to all eighteen piles, but my report was worthless. Foxy was not impressed. It was now midday, and we should have been long finished.

Since Woody had instructed us not to bring food and Verne's fussiness barred provisions on the yacht (though he managed a cup of soup for himself) everyone was starving. With one exception. Me. I was too wet and cold to give a damn about nourishment. I only wanted to finish the job and get the hell out of there.

Foxy came on the phone. "Kirby, go to the offshore pile. I'm going to lower the steel piling straps and the swell indicator from a skiff. Bolt it on at mid-water, about fifteen feet off the bottom."

The straps were very large, large enough to accommodate the three-foot-diameter steel piles, and I told Foxy I could not blow up the needed fifteen feet to bolt them on, much less lift the device in place to do so.

"Okay, dammit," Foxy yelled. "We'll hold them up with a rope and then you bolt them on. Do you think you can do that?"

"I'm sorry," I told him. "I can't blow off the bottom."

"Alright. We'll lower a descending line to you. Do you think you can climb a rope?" Foxy's temper was getting short.

I did my best and barely managed to hang on in mid-water. My hands were busy with the line, and my legs were too rigid to straddle the pile. When I struggled to tie a loop in the end of the line, my foot got caught. The task went on forever. Holding on with one hand, I attempted to juggle wrenches, nuts, and bolts with the other. By three in the afternoon, I was finished with the task, both physically and mentally. Now all I had to do was climb back aboard the *Aquarius* without pissing off Verne. I knew I was a dead man before I started.

His Jacob's ladder, a device designed by the devil, had rope sides and wooden rungs. Climbing one in the dry is difficult; the ladder was floating around on the surface like flotsam. I did my best to pull it down and get my feet on the lower rung but, because I couldn't bend my knees, this simple act took ten minutes.

Once I was mounted on the rope and wood monstrosity, I began doing pull-ups. My feet supported me between each effort but, again because of my stiff non-bending knees, my feet couldn't aid in my advance. The Mark V rig weighed over 150 pounds and, once I began to clear the surface, this was added to the weight of the water in my dress. My legs ballooned with water. I weighed far too much to do anymore goddamned pull-ups; it was all I could do to just stand and hang onto the stupid rope ladder.

Swinging back and forth, my black rubber galoshes were marking and scratching the sides of Verne's light gray showboat. Willie got a rope under each of my arms and the three of them — Woody, Willie, and Foxy — began hauling me up. Verne stood well back in order to avoid soiling his uniform. Once I was high enough, my crew was able to remove my helmet and weight belt. This was a true blessing, but I still had to climb aboard with my legs full of water and unbending knees.

When my waist was higher than the deck, the Jacob's ladder swung out and dumped me, chest first, on the yacht where my brale wing nuts dug divots in the deck. Even worse, they had to dress me out in this embarrassing position, lying face down in an inch of now-contaminated water — the capacity of my bladder having been exceeding during my long ordeal. (For this, I received no sympathy.) Of course Verne was horrified by what I had done to his beautiful deck, what with the dents and the pee.

According to Woody, he had never been in a situation where his dress was too small. He couldn't understand my problem; consequently, he made no excuses to Russell Fox on my behalf. Once I was back in my street clothes, Foxy assured me I was a great hand topside, "but please never show up as a diver on a job of mine again."

As time went on, Foxy related the story to others, including the Associated Divers team. This haunted me for years and later, when I did my best to get on as a diver with Associated, I was refused.

With the exception of Woody, no one wanted me in the water. Woody kept me on under one condition; he insisted I rebuild some of his old helmets that were trashed. I ended up a white helmet slave.

Woody and Meribeth took a two-week vacation, leaving me as the duty diver and Willie as my tender. Chances were, no one would call during their absence, but God has strange ways and one day the phone rang. It was Alex, Tony Metson's nephew. He was now a big wheel with the Cuss Group, a new offshore drilling company. The conductor pipe connected to their underwater well head had been damaged, and its top had to be removed. They had determined that underwater burning was the way to do it and, since Treen's Commercial Diving had been doing their work, I was their man.

Alex came to our mobile home. "Kirby," he said, "this one is a bear. There's only one-quarter-inch clearance between the casing and the conductor pipe inside. We need to cut away the casing, but we can't have one nick on the inner pipe or it will cost us over two million to repair. Can you guarantee success?"

He was leaving it up to me. If I took the job and nicked the pipe, Woody would never get another job with the up-an-coming Cuss Group. If I turned it down, Woody might lose his customer to Associated Divers. I had to make up my mind that minute. My only experience with underwater burning had been in the navy's diving school. This being the case, I declined the job.

Alex called Associated Divers who, with the exception of Laddie, did not have anyone available. Laddie, who had never done any underwater burning, didn't tell them this. Though Lad burned holes here and there, failing to cut the casing free, he did not damage the inside pipe. Art Broman relieved Lad, and was able to complete the task.

When Woody returned, he was irate. He fired me and I returned to my work as a welder and pile driver man for another extended time in my life.

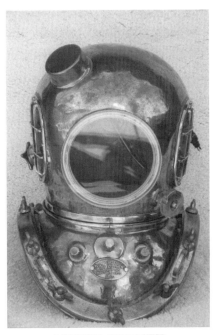

MORSE HELMET

135

The phone rang. "It's Woody," Claudia shouted. "He wants to hire you again."

"Kirby," Woody said, "I just bought an old Morse commercial helmet that needs rebuilding. If you do it, I'll split dive with you on an underwater well completion off the drilling ship *SM-1*." Claudia and I really needed the money so I agreed.

This poor old hat had seen better days. It was too tall — the view port was in line with my forehead. Massive surgery would be required to fashion it into a working helmet. I approached Mr. Treen with a deal. "Look, Woody, the helmet is going to require a couple of weeks work. I'll do it if you let me wear the thing instead of one of those horrible Mark Vs you seem to love."

We shook on it. For the first time, I would have good equipment and might be able to accomplish a handsome amount of underwater, mechanical work.

The job would require four days of around-the-clock diving in one hundred feet — just right for making money; lots of it. We arrived aboard the drill ship as the sun passed downward into the purple horizon. It would take us all night to hook up the completion before it could be pressure-tested, our first step with the long task.

I went to work with Willie, setting up our gear. When I finished, I went back to Woody to have a meeting. He was already in his dress and on the dive stool, wearing the Morse breastplate. I was once again stuck with the damned Mark V.

I was the first in the water where I was to set the twelve-ton stack onto the conductor pipe. This massive rig was lowered by the ship's drilling string. The slight rise and fall of the *SM-1* allowed me to align the mating halves and then have them lowered at just the right moment. I soon had the Cameron clamp in place and tight. The completion was ready for pressure-testing, and everything came off without a hitch. I was proud of my work as I came up and began my in-water decompression stop at forty feet.

By the time I emerged from the decompression tank, the pressure testing was complete. Woody was tasked to install as much of the plumbing as possible before his bottom time was consumed.

Heaving and grunting, he provided us with a vivid account of his progress. "All that remains is for Kirby to tighten it up," he said. "Everything is in place." These words have burned in my mind since. Once he had finished his in-water stop and was in the chamber, I dressed into the Mark V and went down.

I turned on the underwater light. *Nothing* was in place. All the pipes and valves were lying on the hard mud bottom, and our tools were scattered about. Woody had accomplished nothing except to make a mess. I began by rounding up the bag of tools. Then I had to locate the annulus valve and gather its associated piping.

Inserting this component was difficult. The two production lines had to be spread by pulling on them with "come-alongs" before the valve and its respective pipes could be inserted and secured. Each flange required eight bolts and, as I was tightening them, the tool pusher's voice came over my phones. "Hey, diver, what the hell is the matter? Woody told me the annulus valve was in place and ready to be tightened. What's taking you so damn long?"

If I told the truth Mr. Treen would fire me, so I elected to fib. "The tightening sequence of the bolts is very difficult and requires a lot of time. I'm almost finished." I soon had the tools back in their canvas bags and was ready to come up. I was five minutes over my bottom time.

As I sat on the pipe bar counting, "one potato, two potato, three potato..." I felt like a human fishing lure as I was jigged up and down by the motion of the *SM-1*. Each potato was a second, and I had over an hour of decompression before being admitted into the warm, decompression chamber – a hell of a lot of potatoes – with nothing else to do but think about Mr. Whitefish who was probably still looking for me.

Suddenly, I felt a sharp pain in my right shoulder. I had been hit with the bends. Rather than discuss my situation with Willie, I asked to be dropped back down. At sixty feet, the pain went away. After ten minutes, I began to work my way upward very slowly. In an hour I was back at the bar and I resumed normal decompression.

By the time I was back on deck, I was all but frozen. I had, by then, determined that deep water diving was not for me. Inside the chamber, I decided to limit my underwater activities to eighty feet or less, staying within the tables.

When I emerged from the tank I stood face to face with the bad-tempered tool pusher. He advised me to seek employment elsewhere and told me he needed a diver who was a good mechanic, not just a monkey on the end of a hose.

My fib paid off, however, for Woody continued to keep me on, and I was busy for a good year (and yes, I did get to use the rebuilt Morse helmet) setting and hooking up many more well-completions and their associated piping.

At this time, I need to point out that Woody was a particularly fine individual with whom I shared many wonderful adventures. I may have seen him as a poor mechanic, but my hat was always off to him because he more than made up for this as a wonderful businessman. He could secure more contracts with his great personality than any other contractor. I have always wished I were half as good as a mechanic and twice as good a businessman.

Woody brought Treen's Commercial Diving to the top. Then he employed Bud Rogers, another very fine man, as his chief mechanic and together they built an even larger firm.

When they sold the company, they had their equipment painted a metallic blue.

The new owners were less successful, and Woody eventually bought everything back for twenty cents on the dollar. He and Bud repainted all the equipment metallic green before selling it again. We lost track of the number of times the firm was sold; each time this happened the equipment was repainted – metallic blue, then metallic green, then...

The rebuilt Morse hat went to the bottom with a lot of other gear when the *SM-1* capsized and sank during a huge storm off Gaviota.

I only did one more diving job for Woody. That was in 1965 and I cover it in another chapter.

Claudia and I loved Woody and stayed in touch with him after he retired a few years ago. Then, in 1998, he went to the huge decompression tank in the sky.

I hope God didn't plan for him to perform any mechanical tasks.

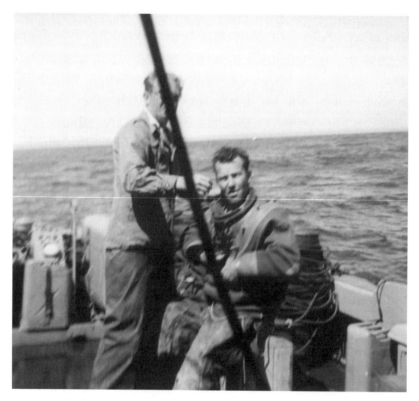

WOODY TREEN

DRIVE A PILE, KEEP A SMILE, AND THE GRIM REAPER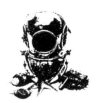

The little wooden barge that the *Rex* and I had smashed into Stearns Wharf ended up anchored in the harbor at Bradley's Reef, her decks awash. Her two low pipe rails, now adorned by countless sea gulls, were the only things visible. The rest of the rig was under water. Bob Forrest, now the barge's owner, had not spent a nickel on it. It would soon sink, becoming a navigational hazard. Hauled off, it would join Greco's Plymouth on Camby's Reef.

I had always wanted a barge. There is something magical about them. They are all business — no show, just go. If I could find a way to put it to use, perhaps I could convince Claudia that we had to have the derelict; it was something every man needed. Easy to see I was no businessman.

An article appeared in the local paper detailing extensive plans for Santa Barbara's new harbor to be built in 1960 and '61. The planned marinas would require many driven piles and, ever since my brief experience with Bob's Sea Foods, I had wanted to drive piles.

Chadwick and Buchanan, heavy-duty builders out of Los Angeles, won the contract and had rented an office in the veteran's building where I had met dredge owner Phillip Ryan years earlier. My introduction to John Buchanan was far different than my encounter with Mr. Ryan, however. Polite, mild mannered and humble, he agreed to hire me when the time was right, but many obstacles remained before the project could begin.

I was off to see Bob Forrest and talk him out of his barge. After I paid him a dollar to legalize the transaction, the barge was mine. Somehow I just <u>knew</u> Claudia would be elated.

Another meeting with John Buchanan and the wheels were in motion. I would repair the old lighter, then turn its keys over as a rather handsome rental. Then I would become his welder, designing and building a pile driver on the decks of the barge. Even better, I would be doing this for union wages.

I had never operated a pile driver; in fact, I knew squat. I was young, fearless, and ignorant. These are the only excuses I can offer for my eagerness.

First I had to repair my submerged vessel, and Joe Greco once again came to my rescue. Securing a line to one corner, we towed the rig into deep water. Then we ran two lines from each far end to the *El Greco's* towing bit. When Joe applied power, my acquisition rolled over as easy as a dog longing to have its belly scratched.

We towed the barge back into the harbor and tied it to the navy pier. Her bottom was now awash instead of her decks.

Two days of standing in the water while removing her sheathing revealed the unfortunate truth. Many planks had been eaten away by shipworms. I would have to stand, kneel, and sit in two inches of water while replacing and caulking the planks. Thank God it was summer and I was young.

I was soaked at the start of each day, and I stayed that way until quitting time. I cut, pounded, and caulked for a week and a half, until the hull was tight. As a diver, I understood something about air pressure. After drilling a hole in her bottom, I screwed a steel pipe into it. Then I ran a rubber hose from this fitting to Bob Benton's diving air compressor on the pier. Soon my pride and joy was floating high and her bottom and sides were drying out. Using fifty gallons of Henry's Roofing Cement as a sealer, I nailed down new plywood sheathing — a trick I had learned while repairing holes in the bottom of the *Paula.*

By the time I was ready to paint her bottom, I was almost out of funds. My puny five gallons of bottom paint would not cover her twenty-by-sixty-foot surface, much less her sides below the water line. A large number of marine bugs thrive in our warm, southern waters, and a protective coating was a necessity. I had to pull another rabbit out of my hat.

This time my rabbit came in the guise of five gallons of the cheapest oil paint produced — with as much lead in it as possible — which I purchased from the Santa Barbara Paint Factory. I mixed the five gallons of paint with five gallons of creosote and as much garden bug killer as I could afford. If I was to create this "mixture from hell" today, the EPA would have me jailed.

After this deadly concoction dried, we flooded the barge again; then Joe and I repeated our offshore drill. I ended up with a decent old scow, and I rented her to John Buchanan the very next day.

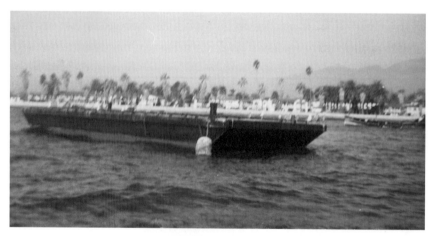

THE BARGE

Everytime I got the chance, I talked with old-time pile drivermen about floating pile driving rigs, and everyone of them had a different method for constructing a pile driver. Emille Guiest, John Buchanan's foreman, wanted greased boards that would slide forward. "Yup," he said, "that's how we did it in the old days — a little slippery but it worked like a charm."

I stopped him short. "Not on my rig," I told him. "There will be no greased cat walks."

An individual then entered my space who changed my life forever. Lloyd Lindwall had been a fisherman and was as tough a man as God ever created. Nothing could stop him. If he didn't know the answer to a problem, he would carry on anyway, leveling everything flat in the process.

If a machine wouldn't start, he would tow it to the ends of the earth in an attempt to reinstall life into its broken heart while seldom addressing the original problem. Lloyd would rip into anything that was assembled with screws, bolts, or welds. If necessary, my hero could probably rip a bowling ball apart with his bare hands.

I had met him for the first time a year earlier at the navy pier when he arrived in what had once been a beautiful, thirty-eight-foot fantail fishing boat. Lloyd's father, who built the boat for Lloyd ten years earlier and had since died, would have probably filled his pants if he had seen her that day, for Lloyd had reduced her to scrap. Instead of wearing her out, he had simply used her up.

As I gazed at the fishing craft, I realized Lloyd had just returned from what appeared to be a very successful fishing trip; one more mackerel would have sunk the boat. Her hold was filled beyond capacity, her decks were loaded, and the engine room was stuffed with oily fish. After a stern speech from Ellen, his wife, he decided to sell what was left of his rig and return to construction work. He had his eyes on the harbor improvement project, and so did I.

Lloyd had worked as a pile driverman in Alaska during the war. John Buchanan could spot a hardworking person and hired him as my assistant. He was soon my close friend and, later, my partner. God, how I loved him! And my goodness, how difficult it was to work with him!

Lloyd helped me complete our pile driver and, each day after quitting time, I would go back and re-weld his work. By the grace of God, the floating rig became a reality without either of us ending up dead in the process.

The day of our first trial is still vivid in my mind. Ken Elms needed a pile driven right in front of the harbormaster's office where everyone could witness our masterpiece — which became known as "Kirby's Folly" — in action. I cringed when Lloyd appointed himself

141

winch operator.

A crowd watched as Lloyd's heavy hand came down on the clutch handle of the winch. I had installed a big V-8, with oodles of oats, from a recently wrecked new Buick. The throttle was wide open, and the long straight exhaust bellowed as the 2000-pound hammer made its rapid journey up the steel leads faster than it could fall.

The steel hoist cable parted when the hammer reached the top pulley and could go no farther. Lloyd had failed to release the clutch lever. The 2000-pound weight then plummeted into the water, resembling a grey whale breaching in search of a mate. The resulting wave of water covered the onlookers as they ran off, laughing.

Don Duckett, owner of a scuba diving shop, came to my rescue by loaning me gear to locate and retrieve the one-ton, cast-iron weight.

Lloyd passed me a manila line which I secured to the hammer, but before I was out of the water and clear, he wound it around the capstan and took a pull. The hammer and follower block caught under the barge's railing, the line parted, and the massive weights just missed me on their way back down.

The following day Mr. Lindwall raised the hammer all the way up and released the clutch, applying full brakes before it fell to the bottom of our steel guides. Once again the stored energy broke the cable and, this time, it pulled down our entire steel structure as well.

Crumpled steel lay everywhere, tangled into a giant, scrap iron pretzel. The hammer and block were back on the harbor bottom as well. My new friend was shouting orders like the skipper of a Mexican tuna boat, while the crowd laughed, cheered, and slapped their thighs. I was mortified.

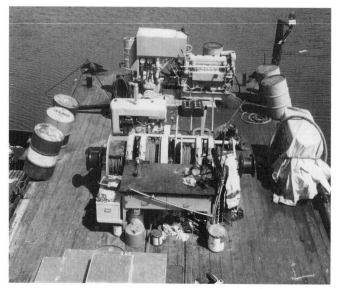

ANCHOR SYSTEM AND PUMP

By the time I had the rig back in order, it was much stronger and I was much wiser. We finally got our "Mutt and Jeff" routine sorted out and began driving piles with a vengeance.

We converted an eighteen-foot skiff into a workboat for moving our barge's 300-pound Danforth anchors. We installed a one-foot-diameter steel pipe through the skiff's center with a small gas-powered winch attached to the upper lip of the pipe. We would fish a crown buoy's cable up through the pipe, secure it to the winch drum, then engage the clutch. The skiff would head straight down for a couple of seconds before the anchor freed itself. Because the anchor now hung below the center of our little work boat, we could easily move the anchor to a new location and drop it again.

Our skiff was powered by a new, forty-horsepower Johnson outboard. In addition to the heavy securing clamps supplied by the manufacturer, the engine was secured to the skiff's transom with two large stainless steel bolts. The mounting appeared to be very strong, but the Johnson company had not allowed for Lloyd Lindwall. One day I heard the skiff coming; Lloyd was shouting but this was not unusual. Then I noticed the two transom bolts were broken, and the clamps were very loose. Lloyd was sitting on the motor, doing his best to hold it down while steering with his butt. I still have no idea how he accomplished this feat or how he had busted up the boat in the first place. But he did.

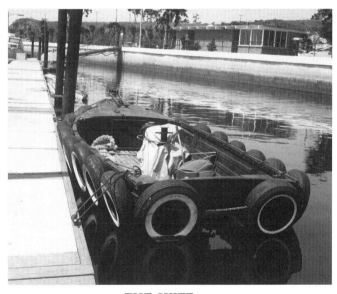

THE SKIFF

Driving piles was fun. Our five-man crew of union "pile butts" were some of the finest men I've ever known. Unfortunately, the wooden piles were pressure-treated with creosote, a mixture of crude oil and acid that has long since been outlawed. When we were downwind of our pile driver's leads, we were sprayed with this toxic mixture with each blow of the hammer. My fair complexion (which usually accompanies those with red hair like mine) could not withstand the acid shower burns nor the sun, and I ended up with a melanoma in the center of my chest. Extensive surgery was required in order to remove the growth.

With the exception of those piles closest to the current launching ramp, the pile driving had been completed by the time I had healed. Because of the harbor's shallow and hard bottom, the piles were unable to penetrate the soil. The harbor would have to be dredged before we could continue. The city, in an effort to save money and face, lent us its small, underpowered dredge, *La Rena*, and her crew. Once a thin layer of sand had been removed, river rocks appeared. Lots of them. We soon learned the entire harbor was lined with the outfall of an ancient glacier. These rocks and our dredge cutter did not get along and, within a week, the dredge crew gave up — right after the four-year-old *La Rena* had done the same thing.

The city then turned to Chadwick and Buchanan who hired a dirt contractor, John Blakemore, to solve the problem. John brought in a very large crawler crane. We anchored the pile driving barge in deeper water and secured a line from the driving barge to a heavy drag bucket which was also attached to the crane's load line. We planned for the crane to pull the bucket in, filled with sand and rocks. Our pile driver would then pull it out. This worked to a degree, but the tough, cobblestone bottom refused to give up much of its terra firma. The bottom was far too hard.

Our next approach was to install a drilling rig on our barge so that we could drill the bottom, load the holes with dynamite, and shoot it. Our intention was to break up the rocks so that the drag bucket could penetrate the loose surface. The drilling and shooting were activities I would pay to do again! We started off with ten sticks of forty percent per hole. This worked but was no big deal, so we upped the load to twenty sticks. This worked better, but each explosion resulted in small, muffled farts that yielded little visual reward. Our Grand Finale was one shot of twenty holes with a case in each. The following day the *Santa Barbara News-Press* reported an earthquake in the harbor area.

God, it was fun! Dead fish were everywhere. My old friend Wayne "Dynamite" Smithson would have creamed his jeans!

If the forty cases of dynamite we had stored in the hull of the barge had ever gone off, the resulting disaster at the waterfront would have put any fireworks display on earth to shame — windows for a half-mile in every direction would have been blown out.

But soon the dredging was completed, and John Buchanan's pockets were lined with dollars from the Santa Barbara City Council's emergency fund.

One more shallow area was then discovered that needed to be removed and, since we had re-tooled for pile driving, we once again reset the drilling rig on deck of the pile driver. Old Charlie, our crane operator from the midwest, was attempting to walk John Buchanan's new QuickWay crane down the launching ramp when it got away from him. "I cain't stop her!" he yelled as he bailed out. The boom swung wildly back and forth, indicating the crane's progress under the surface of the water, before coming to rest with only the upper half of the boom exposed.

Buchanan was fearful his partner, Fred Chadwick, would blow up when he heard about the disaster. His command rang out over the harbor. "Kirby!" he yelled. "Rig up the pile driver and raise my little crane again, and do it soon! Please!"

Lloyd towed over our pile driver, tearing up only a few yachts in the process, and after it was anchored over the crane, I was given the task of rigging the crane underwater for the lift. The only gear I had to work with was my old abalone mask, a hose from my San Diego days, and Bob Benton's compressor.

Commercial diving equipment requires two-way communication with topside for an important reason — it is imperative for adequate safety and efficiency. When I had, earlier, used scuba gear to secure the downed hammer, Lloyd had almost killed me. This was not Lloyd's fault; I was careless and dove in an unsafe manner with improper gear. On the other hand, I could never count on Lloyd to do what I expected or needed; consequently, it was difficult to be sufficiently careful around him. His actions were spontaneous, and he followed through without regard for safety. Understanding this, for reasons I will never know, I dove in gear that did not include two-way communication. Even worse, I would be tended by a man who was unpredictable.

Diving down to the submerged crane, I would feed two heavy steel cables through one set of tracks from the outside. Then I would swim under the crane, between the tracks, and run the cables through the other set of tracks and out the other side. We then planned to hook up these two cables to the load block on our pile driver and lift. When the crane was high enough to clear the three-foot-high concrete lip of the launching ramp, using John Blakemore's large crane, we would pull it back up the ramp.

We loaded Bob's compressor onto a rusted out, engineless "M" boat which was used as a work platform in the harbor. While Joe Greco pulled the "M" boat alongside the pile driver, Lloyd was to tie it off securely.

I made my way underwater and easily ran the cables through the first set of tracks. Making my way under the crane, I squeezed through a narrow opening between the inshore end of the frame of the crane and the three-foot-high cement ramp lip. The offshore end of the crane was buried deep in mud. Once under, I pulled the cables on through, fed them out to the other set of tracks, and headed back to the rather small entrance slot. To my dismay, I discovered the crane had continued to settle, and it looked as if there was no longer enough room for me to make it out. I was suddenly jerked hard against the belly of the crane where I was squashed against the obstructed hole. I had to do something fast, and I took a deep breath and unsnapped my hose from my belt. My mask was jerked off my head and it disappeared through the hole.

Topside, the rusty "M" boat had come untied and was sailing toward the Harbor House Restaurant, trolling my diving mask and hose behind like a salmon lure. Lloyd had failed to tie the boat securely to our pile driver barge.

Now extremely concerned, I turned my head sideways and began to squirm through the tiny opening as quickly as I could. The edges of the rough concrete ramp were cutting into my fresh melanoma scar, but this was the least of my worries. All I could think about was breathing fresh air and, hopefully, seeing my wife again.

Suddenly free, I began ascending without any problems. There, standing on the launching ramp, was John Buchanan. Lloyd, my tender, was missing. "Where the hell is Lloyd?" I shouted.

"Oh," Buchanan answered, "he's in the pickup, going after something."

I swam back to the barge where I struggled to get on deck. Wet and cold, I began to shake. I was then commanded to proceed with the lift. I had once again managed to escape a close encounter with the Grim Reaper.

When Lloyd returned and shouted orders from the cab of his pickup, I gave a sad chuckle. His truck, brand new a year ago when it was entrusted to him, was in worse shape than his fishing boat the day he sold it.

We soon had Buchanan's crane high and dry, but it was very dead. Lloyd calmed down, and we took time to enjoy coffee and laugh about the entire affair. With a little effort, we even got a laugh or two out of Buchanan.

If I had met the Reaper that day, it would have been my own fault. As I said earlier, the dive was poorly organized and all I had to do was say no. My eagerness to help Buchanan was compounded by several foolish blunders, but I lucked out and lived to laugh about them.

Jim Furby, John Buchanan's engineer, and Mario Sotello, a labor foreman, later formed a small pile driving company with Lloyd Lindwall and I. Our company was called Kirby, Furby, Lindwall, and Sotello, and we were amazed by the number of times we were offered jobs in the legal field.

We did secure a large job driving pile in Ventura for the Granite Construction Company. I ran the barge, drove the piling, and spent weekends performing necessary maintenance. After the job was completed and our meager funds were beginning to diminish, the four of us began squabbling like a bunch of biddies in a thrift shop, so we decided to go our separate ways. I ended up with our still-unpaid-for truck crane; my partners took the pile driver and skiff.

From then on no maintenance was done on the rig, and it eventually settled into Ventura's harbor. The entire harbor was later washed out by the river, including the remnants of our rig.

Lloyd and his wife, Ellen, eventually moved to California's Santa Ynez Valley. They remained close to Claudia and I. By the time God took Lloyd in 1989 and Ellen in 1995, they were like a brother and sister to us. How we miss them.

The Chamber Of Commerce

The Chamber of Commerce it might be said
Lies midst the thighs of a woman in bed
Not silver or gold excites or inspires
Like the glance of a lady before she retires

Fortunes are lost and fortunes are made
In the stiff competition of how one gets laid
Businesses thrive or businesses fail
On the prime rate of a prime piece of tail

A man touches death in that glorious spasm
That brings forth new life from that manifold
    chasm
A nation can grow or a people can die
If her legs won't divide, we can't mulitply

So let's have a cheer for that wonderful place
It's the same, no matter the creed or the race
Although I admit that it sounds kind of corny
Try the Chamber of Commerce next time
    you get horny

G.G. Ainsworth

147

OIL, OIL, EVERYWHERE

By 1962 Associated Diver's work invoices had become carte blanche with the offshore drilling companies, creating a cocky mood within their ranks. I can recall Bob Rudi loudly expressing his brash feelings one afternoon: "Damn we're good. If Dan Wilson tries to scoop our deep-water capabilities, I'll bring up his worthless body and personally deliver it to his widow. Associated knows deep diving. The oil companies love us."

At the time it seemed almost impossible for others to break into the petroleum diving field. Nevertheless, some were trying. Two absolutes — nitrogen narcosis and long-in-water decompression limited air diving to 250 feet. The inability to go deeper was holding back offshore development. Frustrated, drilling firms would listen to anyone with a new idea.

Frank, a diver and soldier-of-fortune from Santa Monica, had department heads at Shell Oil listening to claims he could stick his arms through holes in a one-atmosphere bell, sealed with leather at his biceps, and accomplish useful work at any depth. "Oh, it will hurt like hell," he said, "but I can get the job completed. Beyond that, I can dive on Carbagine, a new inexpensive gas I've invented. This stuff is capable of taking me very deep and with no side effects." The Shell troops then realized Frank was full of crap.

U.S. Navy Helium Helmet

Cat. No. 29019

- This is a standard Mark V Model I U.S. Navy Diving Helmet which has been modified in accordance with Navy specifications so as to be usable with helium/oxygen breathing mixtures.

- A canister is mounted on the rear of the helmet, and a venturi re-circulating system uses the canister to scrub CO_2 from the re-circulated gas.

- The breastplate is the same as the standard Mark V breastplate, and all other parts and accessories are inter-changeable except that the standard control valve is modified so that it may be used in the helium mode.

- The canister can be removed, and the inlets from the canister into the helmet can be sealed with brass caps. The helmet is then usable with air and a standard control valve as the equivalent of a Mark V.

- Weight: With canister approximately 93 lbs.

Our U.S. Navy, using helium to replace the nitrogen that caused narcosis, could go deeper than air dives since Swede Momsen's pioneering efforts during the salvage of the *Squalus* in 1939. This, plus later additional naval efforts, was conducted from offshore salvage ships and tugs. After the sinking of the *Squalus*, all ASRs were equipped with heavy mooring systems and escape chambers as per Momsen's mandate.

The navy's converted Mark V recirculator gas saving helmets were cumbersome and heavy. The hat and canister alone weighed 100 pounds, and the remaining rig weighed at least another hundred. An eyelet was fixed to the top of each helmet to facilitate rigging to a block and tackle, the method used to assist the diver to a standing position.

All shipboard gas regulating hardware was also heavy and complex, filling most of the salvage ship with plumbing and chambers. Beyond that, the navy used a toxic chemical, Shell Natron, to scrub the carbon dioxide within their helmets. Natron became lethal if the gear leaked. The navy's method of diving helium was out of the question in our civilian world.

In 1963 Dan Wilson, who was a former abalone diver like me, changed all this by installing a demand regulator inside a light commercial helmet, thus conserving almost as much valuable helium as that conserved with the navy's recirculators. Dan Wilson's helmet was light and simple. Bob Rudi's statement directed toward Dan and his troops accomplished only one thing; by attempting to intimidate Wilson's gang he drove them further and faster, eventually spelling the end for Associated Divers.

Wilson and his new partners, Lad Handelman, Whitey Stefens, Bob Ratcliff and several other individuals also developed a refined gas-regulating box. This portable system was compact enough to lift into a pickup or be placed on the deck of a small boat, and it performed the same task as the naval ASR's complex system. The gas-regulating box was as important a development as Wilson's new helmet.

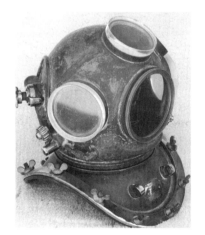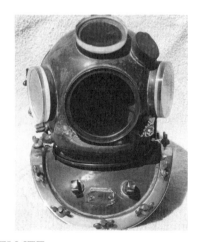

WILSON'S HELMET

149

Their new firm, General Offshore Divers, got its start when they conducted a demonstration dive to over 400 feet in the Santa Barbara Channel, proving they could dive on gas far less expensively than they could when using our navy's system.

Associated Divers, Divcon, and Treen's Commercial Diving knew they were in trouble unless they could break into gas diving as Dan Wilson had done. In order to do this they needed helium equipment, and their only option was to make the helmets and gas regulator equipment themselves. If they failed, their flamboyant lifestyles would come to an end.

Jerry Todd came to our home one summer day in the spring of 1964. "Kirby," he said, "Bob Rudi was dead wrong. Danny's outfit has scooped us. If we don't get into helium, we're dead. Will you design and build us some recirculator helmets? We can pay you $600 a month."

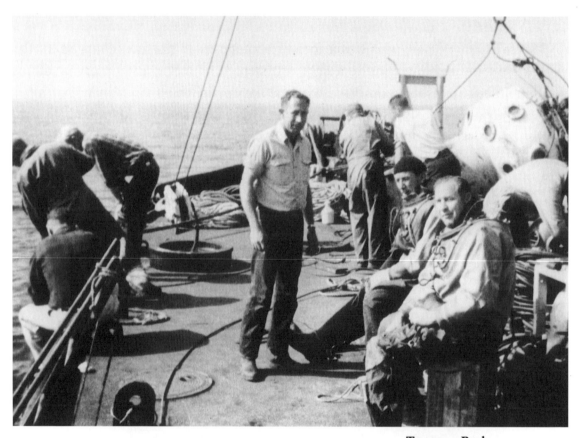

Torrance Pucker
Front: JERRY TODD; middle, TED BENTON; back, TEDDY TODD

I agreed. Having no idea where I might end up, I now entered the commercial diving equipment business. Looking back, my road to fame (and not much fortune), though very interesting, was filled with large cobblestones, deep ruts, and lots of mud. Accomplishing

150

anything worthwhile is not simple!

Associated Divers was founded by Charlie Isbell in 1956, with partners Murray "Blackie" Black and Eldon Smith. Ted Benton, Woody Treen, Jerry Todd, Peter Brumis, Ken Knott, and Bob Rudi would later join the ranks, thereby creating a potent diving team. After a time, Blackie left to found Divecon International; Woody formed Treen's Commercial Diving; and Charlie hung up his diving dress for good. Bob Rudi became salesman for Associated, and he stayed until the company's demise in the fall of 1965.

My first day in their dilapidated office (the antiquated marine corps automotive repair facility at Goleta Airport) was spent in a design meeting with five stockholders and numerous tenders, divers, and friends. During the day, troops appeared, then left. The golf greens held far more appeal than the design of diving helmets, and reality had not yet set in. They were going broke but didn't know it.

Many design possibilities were explored. Murray had designed four recirculator helmets for himself. Each appeared to have a miniature garbage can soldered onto its rear. The rest of us held out for something smaller and more convenient. Holding a Sodasorb canister on the back on a helmet, Ed wondered, "Why can't we do something like this?"

A few simple sketches, and I was off to visit Richard "Dick" Quittner who owned Experimental Machine Shop at the airport. This was the first time I had been involved with this thin machinist. We had a lot to learn about one another − our relationship was probably harder on Dick than it was on me − but we got along amazingly well and established a strong friendship that has lasted over forty years.

My new friend, with flowing brown hair, had apparently been raised on milk toast and tea. Unlike me, he was not a risk-taker − no wild women and no wild, drunken parties. Resourceful and educated, Dick had emerged from the halls of Santa Barbara's University of California as a fire-breathing liberal, while I was a rabid conservative and, like most divers, I was also rather crude. But I understood machinists better than Dick understood divers.

Machinists are exacting and organized and, recognizing Dick's standards, I knew he would always produce a part that was precisely machined. Unfortunately, to Mister Quittner's dismay, I needed loose tolerances.

I told him the threads he had cut into the outside edge of a brass ring, the one that retained the absorbent canister, were not loose enough. "What do you mean 'looser'?" he insisted. "Those threads are just right."

"Bullshit," I said, dropping the ring on the concrete floor and mashing the threads. "Okay, Dick, let's see you thread the son-of-a-bitch together now!" I explained that everything on an oil rig is cold, oily, bathed in salt water, and covered with a thick layer of rust and snot — nothing nice, including its crew. Dick eventually understood the reasoning behind the sloppy machine tolerances required by the diving industry and its uneducated tenders.

Richard became our savior. I presented my ideas, he would make some sketches, and then he would turn out the parts. His designs were wonderfully simple, his machining superb, and he was the most honest man I have ever known.

In a month our first recirculator helmet was completed. It employed a heavily modified, standard navy-style venturi to power our gas in a circle through a canister filled with the non-toxic Sodasorb scrubbing chemical.

The navy gas hat scrubbers were loaded from the outside, and they had to be removed from their respective helmets before they could be filled with the dangerous Shell Natron absorbent. This toxic chemical had severely burned, and in some cases killed, divers when leaks occurred. Because our design loaded a plastic canister from the helmet's interior, our design was far safer, and the helmets were also fifty pounds lighter.

I was introduced to Del Thomason, a retired navy master diver who was an oilfield diver and a very good hand. Del, like me, had been a metal smith in the navy, and I was to assist him in designing and building our new gas control system. Later, after the demise of Associated, Del was employed by Danny Wilson and, within a couple of years, he had designed and built his own recirculator diving helmet. This copper hat was produced by Agonic Machine Shop in Santa Barbara (later known as General Aquadyne) and it was their first attempt to penetrate our market. A single-ported hat, it was not successful. It was eventually given to Whitey Stefens who, following Del's death, gave it to me. After rebuilding the hat, I donated it in 1999 to the Historical Diving Society.

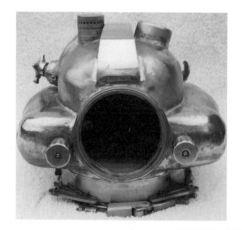 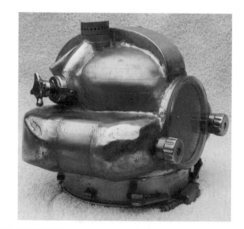

THOMASON'S HELMET

Within two months, Del and I had our first large, steel, chest-style manifold completed. It was outfitted with three volume tanks and pressure reduction valves, all large enough to run the same system that was used aboard the ASRs on which Del had served. His navy programming would not allow him to accept the simple design that had been worked out by Whitey Stefens whom many considered to be a rogue designer. Were they ever wrong!

Preparing for our initial sea trials, all we had to do was pressure our oxygen system. We turned on this gas and stood around, listening for leaks. The steel box then burst in an explosion resembling a Roman candle and sounding much like an Atlas Rocket during lift off. Harry Hurston quickly turned off the oxygen supply at the bottle. Several of us were burned including Jack Fonner who was hospitalized. The large steel box melted in half.

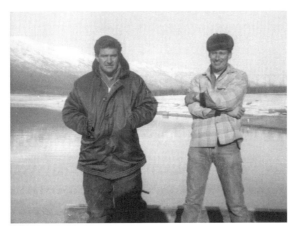

Ed White
L to R: ED WOOD, HARRY HURSTON, 1964

The culprit was a valve that had been sent to us with a "certified clean" label but still contained oil. The explosion was the result of pressurized oxygen coming in contact with the oil. We were left with a healthy respect for oxygen and oil. Ken Knott had also been a master diver in the navy during the war, and he and Del lectured us concerning the cleaning of internal parts. After rebuilding the gas control box, we were again ready for sea trials.

We had six hundred feet of hose coiled over each side of a steel pipe frame, one connected to the experimental helium helmet and the other to a standard air hat as a standby which was plumbed to gas as well. Our gas source was two six-packs of high-pressure helium and oxygen mix. We loaded it onto the deck of Ken Elms' steel supply boat, the *Packer*. Ted Benton was our test diver, Kenny Knott was our standby diver, and the rest of us were helping or tending.

153

Ted spent his maximum bottom time at three hundred feet and, after suffering no carbon dioxide buildup, proclaimed our helmet to be a success. I was instructed to build five more hats for a total of six gas rigs — Associated's passport to success. Or so we thought at the time.

All hats were built on Desco sponge-helmet frames. The first hat had thin plastic view-port lenses and the last five had one-inch-thick plastic screw in ports — a far safer design and one I would continue to use in future Kirby Commercial Helmets.

Once we had completed and tested the first hat, I determined the navy's method of pumping gas through the absorbent could be improved. I turned the entire system around so that, instead of pushing the gas, the venturi would pull the gas through. This proved to be far more efficient.

Bob Rudi promised us lots of work, but it never materialized. I could never understand how his fellow shareholders justified his $3,000 a month wage — the equivalent of $12,000 today. The fee did not include his equally staggering expenses.

Rudi did not sell one job. Instead, he spent his time on the golf course, riding in a jet, or in some bar charming the underpants off females — a noted ability.

He eventually secured a job out of Anchorage in the Cook Inlet. It was to begin in two months, so we crammed gearboxes to their limits and jammed a chamber full of gear including two sets of our new helium equipment — all to be sent to Alaska. Everyone was smiling as the commercial trucks pulled away; I stood by, scratching my head and wondering why helium gear would be needed in the shallow inlet.

Rudi informed us that, in order to secure more work, an office was needed in Anchorage. He bought a large home overlooking the city and Cook Inlet, changed the name of the company from Associated Divers to Associated Divers of Alaska, and we never saw Rudi or the gear again.

The squabbling began, and our funds soon dried up. Jerry loaned the corporation money, but it wasn't enough to sustain us for long. Very soon, it became apparent that Associated Divers was in financial trouble. The arguments were always over the same issue — union membership and union pay scales. The troops at Associated were in Pile Drivers Union 2375 and wanted their accustomed pay rates to continue. Dan, Lad and Whitey had never belonged to a union and saw no sin in charging whatever they wished, causing the oil companies to receive that warm and fuzzy feeling that accompanies a good deal. The past good work done by Associated was forgotten in an instant.

The new generation of oil company production whiz kid managers had replaced folks like Russell Fox, and these young men had a different philosophy about bidding and awarding jobs. A reputation for doing good diving work soon meant nothing; the days of carte blanche were over and would never return. Price had become the only criteria, and it still is. Even worse, our latest generation of managers have even sharper pencils.

The issue of union rates was never resolved. Jerry wanted to scrap them, Ken and Pete wanted to maintain them, and Ted Benton was willing to go with the majority. Arguments became bitter. Jerry threatened to load up most of the remaining gear and drive it to the gulf if his loan was not repaid.

And one Sunday morning he did just that. Ed Wood drove the loaded '49 Chevy flat-rack that towed the chamber; Jerry departed Associated's facility in his pickup. I didn't see Jerry again for a long time, but Ed was back soon. He hated Morgan City, Louisiana, and who could blame him? This gulf coast town was no Santa Barbara! Instead, the culture revolved around swamps, decaying cypress trees, venomous snakes, and overweight ladies minus teeth; it did not revolve around a warm ocean, palm trees, and bikini-clad beauties.

On the Monday following Ed and Jerry's departure, Associated's galvanized metal building was rather empty. The office furniture, such as it was, remained, plus two air hats and miscellaneous parts that were sitting in plywood gearboxes. One well-seasoned compressor, covered with spider webs, sat in a corner. A ladder constructed of re-bar and some worn-out rope hung over large spikes protruding from an open-studded wall. A rusty chamber was outside the building; it had been hurriedly removed from its trailer (also missing) the morning of Jerry and Ed's departure.

We had our final meeting. Pete Brumis had inherited the corporation so he would buy the remaining equipment; Ken Knott and Harry Hurston planned to go to Los Angeles to seek construction diving work; and Ted and Bob Benton planned to work whenever they could for whomever they could.

Bob Rudi, who was becoming very wealthy, hit a non-movable tree in a snow mobile accident and was killed. By the time Associated's helium equipment was discovered in Alaska, it had become obsolete.

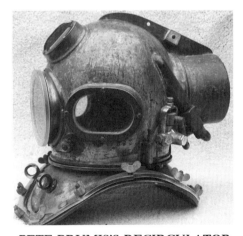

PETE BRUMIS'S RECIRCULATOR

I rented a shop in even worse shape than the tin structure that had once belonged to Associated – and right next door. With the blessings of all, I began producing my line of Kirby Commercial Helmets – both recirculators and air hats. My first customer was Pete Brumis who needed a gas hat, since all six of the others had gone to the winds. I assembled his hat out of scrap parts; Pete had to be one of the cheapest men on earth.

The hat is on display in the Santa Barbara Maritime Museum today. Each time I walk by it, I marvel at the frugality of its now-deceased owner, a man I learned to love.

A couple of years later Jerry Todd sold his fledgling gulf firm to Ocean Systems, founded by and owned, in part, by Dan and Whitey who had split from Lad and his new firm, Cal Dive. Dan eventually sold out and then founded Sub Sea International which he ran for many years before retiring.

Lad ended up merging Cal Dive with Can Dive of Canada, and World Wide Divers of Morgan City, forming Oceaneering International – the world's largest diving organization at that time.

Sometime later, before retiring, he re-organized Cal Dive and built a beautiful home overlooking the entire City of Santa Barbara. Lad turned out to be the most successful of us all. Then misfortune reared its ugly head, for he was injured in a ski accident and ended up a quadriplegic.

We often get together to talk about the "old days." I assist Lad with the continuing problems with his wheelchair, while he does his best to instill some sort of business understanding into my thick skull, mostly a waste of his time.

During the early days of gas diving, though we were doing our best to catch up with Dan Wilson, we never did. He and his gang were a swarm of locusts, marching along – hot on the heels of a new type of diving system that we had only heard of – saturation diving. Dr. George Bond, a navy captain who became known as the father of saturation diving, had conducted experiments at the U.S. Naval Submarine Research Laboratory in the fifties. These tests confirmed the practical application of J.S. Haldane's turn-of-the-century decompression theory; once a diver's tissues become completely 'saturated' with gas, his later decompression requirement will be the same, regardless how much time is spent at that depth.

Bond's efforts spurred the next phase of commercial saturation diving and, in 1964, Wilson and his troops produced a saturation bell called the *Purisima*. We heard words of this new adventure over the bamboo telegraph.

The system had three balls, each about five feet in diameter, and mounted over one another in a stack resembling a large, bright, orange sign over a pawnshop. The top ball was a buoyancy tank. An observer was housed at one atmosphere in the center ball or bell.

Should the need arise, this chamber could then be equalized with the bottom bell.

A diver was to be blown down to bottom pressure in the bottom bell so as to exit and work while the man in the middle bell observed. If the diver needed assistance, the observer would equalize pressure, drop out, and help. This was the theory, at least.

Ultimately, the *Purisima* was not a success, but General Offshore Divers learned enough to build the next generation of larger-diameter, single-sphere bells that did work.

Construction on the *Purisima* took place during the meltdown of Associated Divers. Even though we were on opposite teams, we continued to share a sense of humor and an admiration for one another. We were always trying to come up with a way to have some fun while getting at Danny. After putting on my thinking cap, I came up with a bright idea.

Calling upon my buddy, Joe Greco, I borrowed an old net buoy. These spheres were made of light steel and they were about the same diameter as Dan's bell. We painted ours signal orange – the same color as the *Purisima* – and printed THE PERSIMMON in bold, black letters on its side. I called Del to let him in on our ploy. "Tell Wilson Associated Divers has their new bell completed and ready for sea trials."

Soon, Dan and his troops, arriving in two cars, parked out of sight behind an adjacent hanger. We peeked out of all available holes, watching Dan's team doing the same thing behind the hangers. One at a time, and very slowly – like foot soldiers in a war maneuver – they began to creep forward. Everyone, with the exception of Dan, was in on the gag, and once he was close enough to realize our latest and greatest bell system was actually an orange net buoy, the rest of us came out of hiding to greet one another, slap our thighs, and laugh our butts off.

Everytime I run into Dan these days, he brings up our ploy. It was great fun and an excellent testimony to all of us and our chosen profession. What a wonderful group of free-thinking people, and what an exciting chapter in diving history!

Looking back, I realize Associated Divers had no chance. Wilson and his men were advanced thinkers and able to look far into the future. Beyond that, they were willing to spend the painful effort to get there, something Associated's troops would not do. It is tough to beat a team like that. I feel honored to have known them.

R. KIRBY, COMMERCIAL HELMETS

I enjoyed being at the airport, smelling the aviation fuel and listening to the roar of the huge engines as they ran up, belching blue smoke. Flying machines were my second love; diving my first. Nevertheless, in order to make a living, I had to distance myself. Aviation would have to wait for another time.

I eventually constructed many gas and sixteen air hats, all adorned with a diamond nameplate reading: "R. Kirby, Commercial Helmets."

I initially built an air hat for myself, complete with bells and whistles. Someday I might be offered another diving job and, if I had my own hat, I would never have to dive another Mark V. I continued to be haunted by memories of my experiences with Woody and his worn-out gear.

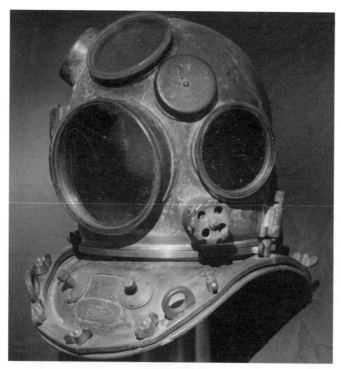

ORVILLE

My new hat, like all those that came after, was built on a Yokohama breastplate. I purchased these, new, for $250. My copper dome was spun by Hummel Sheet Metal in Santa Barbara. With the exception of the air control valve supplied by Morse, Dick Quittner machined all the hardware, and I eventually abandoned the Morse valve for a

158

valve Dick designed for me.

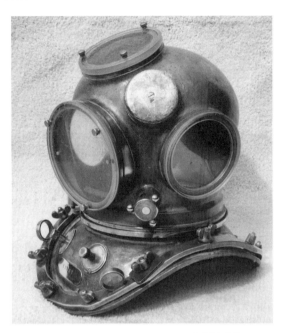

KIRBY AIR HELMET, ORVILLE

The completed helmet was just what I wanted; for the time being, anyway. As a way of life, I would regularly change my mind and make modifications. Innovations came to me daily and often depended upon my mood. I hated the day-by-day manufacturing process − where the actual money is made. I preferred playing around with each new gimmick, tweaking it, turning it over, soldering on a fitting, and then adding air pressure. I had fun building my little air helmet and had no thought of actually selling it. Looking back, I realize this was always a silly approach. I would make a helmet for myself, be forced to sell it, make another, sell it. Anyway, when I finished my first new hat I named it "Orville" in honor of the aviation pioneer, Orville Wright.

I had no sooner completed Orville when an old and dirty 1949 Chevy pickup pulled up in front of my establishment. The pickup sported a fresh brown paint job that had obviously been applied in a hurry with a worn-out paint brush over dirt, dents and rust. Crap was dangling everywhere; shovels, rope, and countless other items indicated that the owner was a miner. A homemade, out-of-square plywood camper had been shoved into the truck's bed, and its poorly hinged rear door was swinging in the breeze, exposing a half-chewed and rotten pack rat's nest within. I would not have been surprised to see Melvin C. Catrel and Three Tit stumble out.

"MUSHY KING, DIVER," according to the letters glued onto the cab's door; inside the cab sat a bushy-haired, bearded, and scroungy-looking man. The door opened slowly and out he climbed, wearing cowboy boots, dirty Levis, and a sweaty western hat. Before he had opened his mouth, I knew another Jim Penn had entered my life; a pseudo-diver who had probably never smelled salt water, much less been immersed in it.

Holding out a callused hand and, using a well-used line, he introduced himself. "Hi," he said, "My name is Mushy. I want you to build me a hat. I'm a diver in San Francisco where men are men and women are darned glad of it."

Without allowing me to get a word in, he continued. "I need a hat designed for dirty water, you know, a small port...hell, no port at all. The water's black, can't see a thing anyway, no used tryin'. Maybe you can keep the price down by not charging me for the things?"

I pointed out that not being able to see in the water was one thing; being blind on deck was something else. But, against my better judgement, I consented to construct a hat with one small Japanese port in front. (Pete Brumis christened it "Cyclops.")

Three weeks later the dingy truck returned and Mushy, happy as a submerged geoduck clam, informed me that he worked for Al Podesta, and he paid me in cash.

A phone call confirmed my suspicions. The San Francisco troops had never heard of Mushy King.

I never heard of him or Cyclops again. I decided Mushy was a Walter Mitty, probably a scuba diver from Nebraska with an itch to move into the sea and, chances are, Cyclops is covered with dust someplace, alongside Mushy's bones in the back of a Nevada mine shaft, awaiting the bewilderment of future archaeologists.

My production line was now well-established, and I received a phone call or two almost every day requesting price and delivery information on air and gas hats. Once a week or so, I would even get a genuine order.

During these good times, every diving contractor wanted to get into the deep-water act. Many had little or no experience with heavy gear, especially the firms in the gulf who were diving Jack Browne masks, with and without communications. They had only one use for gas hats and that was to let the world know they were keeping up with the times. Often as not, my equipment never got wet. Instead, it probably sat in an office for a time, then migrated to a home where it was placed on a stand, thereby providing a nautical touch to the decor.

When saturation diving took over, my orders for heavy gear fell off sharply.

One day, to my surprise, Murray D. "Blackie" Black walked in. Blackie was a former heavy-gear abalone diver who, according to his reputation, did not fear the devil himself. I had met Blackie in the earlier days when we were all rowdy drinkers. He seemed to have a very short fuse then, and he took an immediate dislike to me; in fact, he had threatened − more than once − to punch my lights out. And he was quite capable of doing just that!

Now he was standing in my shop and extending his hand. We shook and have remained friends since.

Dan Wilson had started a chain reaction with his second-generation bell diving system. In order to get into the saturation business before Ocean Systems dominated the entire industry, Divecon International (Blackie's corporation), and all other diving firms were scrambling to construct bells of their own.

Blackie told me he needed four of my heavy recirculator hats rigged so he could dress himself within the confines of his proposed saturation bell. He was confident he could then swim out to his underwater job sites.

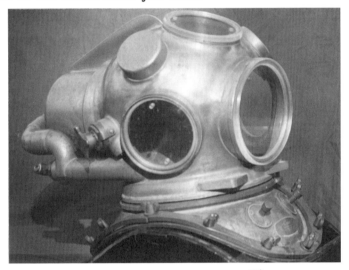

Divecom
MURRAY BLACK GAS HAT

As a rule, saturation diving bells are anchored in midwater, not on the bottom, and divers have to be able to swim — something most divers in heavy gear cannot do. Dan Wilson was the first to address this problem. He hired two abalone divers, Pat Kern and Bev Morgan, to build a diving mask similar to the abalone gear used in southern waters. His mask differed in that it was constructed of fiberglass instead of metal and, to save gas, a demand regulator was incorporated.

Murray Black saw bell diving in a slightly different light. Recognizing the primary need was to keep the diver warm while retaining communication topside, he elected to use heavy gear despite its not being user-friendly while swimming.

Dan Wilson had underestimated the need for communications and for keeping the diver warm. His thin wet suits and leaky dry suits were hopelessly inadequate; obstacles that had to be eliminated before bell diving and saturation diving could become practical techniques.

I questioned Blackie concerning his method of dressing himself in. "Oh hell, Kirby," he said, "I don't mean the breastplate, just the hat. I need two metal plates with holes in them soldered onto the helmet's neck ring. Inside the bell I'll have two large screen door latches. I'll drop these two hooks into the holes on my hat so I can screw myself into the rig. Don't worry, I can swim like mad in heavy gear."

I had no reason to question Blackie's swimming capabilities; my concern was for his other divers. "Oh, well," I told myself, "the customer is always right."

I completed the four recirculators, lined them up against my new pickup, and took a photograph for posterity. Then Blackie picked them up and paid me $1300 each, all in cash.

I didn't mention the transaction to Claudia. I planned to use the nest egg for the business, not on food, Kotex, mortgage payments, and other "unnecessary" items, and I suspected she wouldn't understand.

My telephone fell silent. The market for heavy gear dried up overnight with only three exceptions: J. Ray McDermott & Co. of New Orleans wanted a gas hat; J. & J. Diving of Pasadena, Texas, needed one; and Del Thomason ordered one for Ocean Systems.

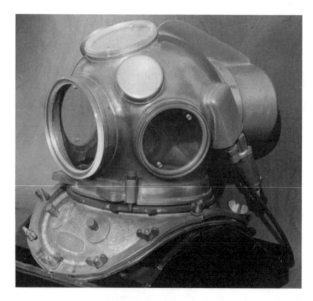

KIRBY GAS HAT

Del's phone call had me confused. Why weren't they using their own system, the demand valve, inside their helmets? After Del picked up the hat, I waited for a second order which never came. I discovered the reason for Del's order later. Dan, Del, and Whitey had split from Laddy and Cal Dive, forming Ocean Systems. They needed good deep-water capabilities and our designs were the best. In an effort to spend less on the helmets, Del took ours to Japan where it was copied by Yokohama Diving Apparatus. I knew chances were good the three helmets I had just sold would be my last commissions in copper and brass. In order to survive, I once again needed to pull that rabbit out of my hat.

In order not to flounder, I had to educate myself in the making of fiberglass masks and helmets. I drove to the breakwater where I sat on the concrete wall, gazing at the fishing boats while drinking coffee and pondering my next move.

As luck would have it, Bev Morgan was standing on the navy pier. Because of Dan Wilson's success with the masks Bev Morgan and Pat Kern had built, I had heard a lot about Bev, but I had never met him. He was not a tall man but, as a result of many years surfing, he had a powerful chest – as if he might crush tires for a hobby. And I had never seen such large arms. I introduced myself. "I'm Bob Kirby," I told him. "I need to hire you to design and construct a fiberglass mask."

He was very polite but informed me he was in no position to take time off, for he was in debt and had to make another abalone trip or he would lose his home.

My roll of bills got his attention. We walked to a nearby coffee shop where he accepted my offer of $600, in advance, for a month's work. We would make a short run of fiberglass abalone masks, then move towards commercial construction masks. That is, if all went well and my money held out.

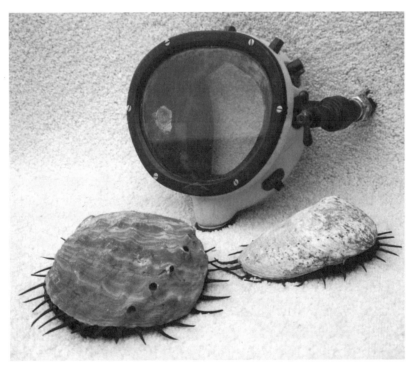

ABALONE AIR MASK, 1965

163

We labored very hard. Bev Morgan was as hard a worker as anyone I had ever known and, even more important, the two of us were compatible in the shop environment. He cleaned up after himself and was thoughtful of others. It was a wonderful month, and we ended up with a production abalone mask that was better than anything on the market.

Major changes took place during our second month together. First, we had to finish the three gas hats McDermott, J. & J., and Ocean Systems had ordered; second, I asked Bev to become my partner and he accepted.

I taught him how to solder copper and brass helmets together; he was an eager student. He, in turn, taught me how to make hand-shaped plugs and molds for fiberglass. We continued as a great team for three more years, designing and producing the most advanced diving equipment in the world under our new nameplate: "Kirby Morgan Corporation."

The money was always tight. I glanced at Orville everyday, sitting beside my desk, waiting to get wet and provide a financial shot in the arm. More important than the money, I still loved to dive.

Woody Treen called one day to tell me about a one-month shallow water job in Eureka and promised a handsome check. Bev and I agreed; the money was too good to turn down, and it was important for me to say current with my diving. I would take a leave of absence while he continued to work on our current project, designing a mask for both commercial and sat diving. This would become our first commercial mask design.

Before I took off, Walt Swenson, an abalone mask customer, walked in with a small complaint. His face was black and blue, his eyes were red balls mounted in the rear of black tunnels and, mad as hell, he was looking for a fight. He addressed Bev first — thank goodness for that. My street-wise partner folded his arms and listened, gigantic triceps swelling and throbbing, as Walt spit out words such as "kill" and "dead."

Walt's story unfolded. His hose had been ruptured at the compressor, the non-return valve had failed and, with the resulting squeeze, his eyeballs had been pulled out of their sockets and had ended up resting on his cheeks. As a last resort before dying, he had relieved the vacuum by breaking out the safety glass port with his abalone bar, and he had almost drowned in the process.

According to Walt, his tender then covered Walt's head with a gunnysack and continued to throw buckets of water on it until they reached the Santa Barbara dock. "That's all I can do for you," the doctor said, popping Walt's eyes back into their sockets.

Once Walt had calmed down, Bev took the mask into our shop and pulled apart the non-return valve. It was filled with rubber cuttings from hose ends that had been improperly installed. Walt had caused the problem himself, and he had almost died.

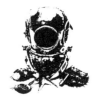

HEALY TWO BITS

The job Woody had phoned about was for Healy Tibbetts Construction Company, a large San Francisco company that had been awarded an outfall extension by one of the Eureka pulp mills. It was to take place that summer, 1965. Woody had agreed to rent them the needed diving equipment and provide them with a list of divers who knew pipe work. The firm asked Hughie Hobbs and me to do the diving, and we accepted.

I loaded Claudia, our two small sons, and my gear into my pickup. My gear included Orville, thank God. Willie had loaded Treen's Commercial Diving pickup with as much junk equipment as they could bill to the Healy job, including their terribly Mark Vs. The better equipment was reserved for the more lucrative work offshore where Woody himself would be diving.

Our equipment was being loaded onto the work boat when I arrived at Eureka's harbor pier. At one time, Woody's diving air compressor, powered by a German Deutz diesel, had been a decent machine. In order to hide its now-sad condition, it had been painted a shiny metallic green. No serious maintenance had been performed, and the engine oil looked like Bunker C found in the bottom tanks of a freighter. The oil filter was heavy, indicating a large volume of dirt within. If we expected the engine to survive the six-week project, we would have to change the oil and get rid of the contaminated filter.

Eureka was not the place to re-locate exotic German machinery. Woody agreed to ship us a filter but, until it arrived, we would have to make do. Unfortunately, it never arrived.

The steel work boat took us the four miles to the Healy Tibbetts derrick barge. From a distance it had appeared quite small, but as we drew closer we were astonished at its actual size. It was more than adequate for the task of extending the thirty-six-inch steel and concrete outfall pipe another five hundred feet. The barge, *Healy Tibbetts No. 7*, was a black steel rig, perhaps ninety feet in length, outfitted with a very large fixed stiff-legged crane. It contained perhaps five feet of freeboard, just enough to keep its decks dry in the northern California sea. Hank, the crane's operator, sat in a control cab halfway up the high A-frame where he enjoyed a bird's-eye vantage point.

Hank, a large man, had white hair, wore a baseball cap, and probably knew as much about offshore crane work as any man alive. His talented hands never moved a lever unless the order to do so was sane and proper.

This was the first time I had worked with Hughie Hobbs. It wasn't long before I knew he was not only a gentleman, but also a very good diver. All tending would be done by two of the pile drivermen already on board. I had my reservations about this until I learned the two men were Pierre Seine and Verne Goldwater. Pierre and Verne had once worked with me as welders on the assembly of a small offshore oil jacket in Long Beach, and I've never known men of better caliber. (Pierre recently retired as the business agent for Local 2375 Pile Drivers Union while Verne went on to become an attorney. Poor bastard.)

Hughie, himself, was a wonderfully mild-mannered man who started out in the abalone patch as a Black Fleet diver. At one time he owned the *Whirlaway* with Ralph Eder. While abalone diving, Hughie and I had been educated on the ways of the sea. We had commanded our own boats, hired our own crews, and solved the many problems only an abalone diver would encounter. Self-reliant, we had learned how to handle people and tight situations. Unfortunately, what we were about to encounter was not merely another tight situation but a political nightmare. We were ill-prepared for what lay ahead.

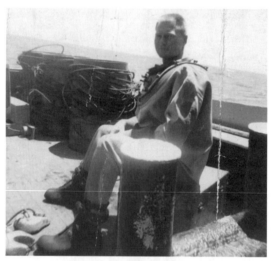

KIRBY, DRESSED IN

Every man on the crew was as good as they come with one exception; Del De Witt who was our foreman. Del was from Oklahoma where deep water was non-existent. The closest he had ever come to the type of work we were supposed to accomplish was laying an irrigation pipe in a ditch. He was, however, a very close friend − possibly even a relative − of the Healy superintendent, Norm Jones.

Norm had spent his life working on the water; at one time he had even been a diver, and he was aware Del knew nothing about offshore construction. Norm had planned on being there to assist Del and possibly mold him into a better kind of man. If, for any reason, Norm was not nearby, Del was an accident waiting to happen.

Our task was tough. The barge *Healy Tibbetts No. 7* was anchored in forty feet of water. On this particular stretch of the Northern California coast, the seas normally run with vigor. Even though we were a half-mile offshore, the swells were high and the water moved fast. These upheavals caused the barge to run in, then out, with great speed and authority. The anchor wires actually sang their complaints, snapping and popping as they were stretched to their limits. With the exception of Del, all of us were in constant fear of an anchor wire breaking while we were latched to equipment on the bottom. If this should occur, there was a good chance the pipe might be damaged. We could even lose a diver.

The bow of the barge was covered by a giant stack of cement-coated steel pipes; each pipe was thirty feet long and weighed fifteen tons. Sitting behind the stack was a pipe-laying "horse," a steel rectangle, twenty-three feet long and fifteen feet wide. It rested on four hydraulic telescoping legs that were fifteen feet high.

Riding on rails and wheels that sat just under this huge rectangle was a smaller rectangle that could be moved front, back, or sideways with hydraulic rams that were controlled by a manifold of valves on deck. Jim Orland, our operator, had been involved in the conception of this monster, and he could make it talk. The little man with the wavy white hair was also a prince.

When we were rigging to set a pipe joint, the horse was positioned over a single pipe on deck with the crane. Two slings were then passed under each end of the pipe and their looped ends were secured to the smaller mobile frame. The entire thirty-five-ton assembly was then lifted and swung over the barge's stern.

Two spar buoys tied to each end of the previous section indicated its location and alignment. Hank had to position the horse and then lower it forty feet to the bottom and a safe distance away – perhaps three feet from the last pipe flange.

This was very difficult as the large swells were continuously raising and lowering the load as the waves of water traveled under the barge's hull. The extreme length of the stiff leg boom amplified the swell, triggering even more problems and white knuckles. Hank had to wait for just the right moment to set the horse onto the ocean floor. Then a diver would enter the water and proceed to the flanged joint that was to be made up. As a rule, there was either very little visibility – or no visibility at all.

While giving verbal directions to Jim at the control manifold, the diver guided the pipe into place by feel while carefully keeping his hands out of the path of the swinging fifteen-ton pipe. This was not a game for children.

Once we had set up our equipment, I dressed in. Using Orville for the first time, I descended to inspect the flow diffuser that was bolted on the end of the existing outfall in order to determine what problems would be involved in its removal.

As I left the deck I heard a disturbing metal-on-metal screeching from within our compressor but, deciding there was nothing we could do about it since we had already changed its oil, I put it at the back of my mind.

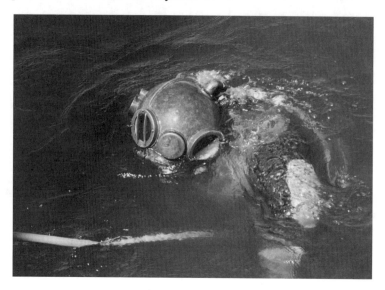

HUGH HOBBS

The diffuser was buried to one-third of its height in the sandy bottom, and it took me an hour and a half to jet it clear and loosen the eighteen one-inch bolts securing it to the last flange on the end of the outfall. I then came up and Hughie relieved me.

Orville was proving to be a wonderful helmet. It was comfortable, displayed excellent balance, and the field of view from the one-inch-thick front port was fantastic. When I could see, that is. As I mentioned earlier, most of the time in these northern waters, I could not see anything.

I was thankful the helmet ports were strong for, in the past, the motion of the running seas had driven me into steel objects with horrific force. The old-fashioned glass ports would have failed me.

The diffuser was soon on deck and the day was used up. Hughie came up, and we dressed out. We would make our first joint the following day, and Norm was pleased. We went ashore, and I had a beer before joining my family in the small motel room we had rented.

I had a difficult time sleeping that night. Recalling the screeching sounds from the compressor, I was concerned. Downtime on a rig is very costly and, should the compressor fail, chances are Woody's gear and two divers would be put ashore.

168

Our first attempt to set a pipe joint was jinxed. Before we could rig the pipe we had to clean up our working space on deck.

As Hank came back on his hoist lever to pick up one of several large anchor crown buoys, Norm suddenly appeared and, before Hank could see him, the heavy can swung into our superintendent with a crushing force, leaving him with a concussion and five broken ribs. Now, instead of tutoring Del as planned, Norm would be spending the next three weeks in a Eureka hospital. The entire crew recognized this as an ominous turn of events, but we could do nothing to change it.

Once Hank had placed the horse on the bottom, because I had an easy time determining direction on the bottom, it was decided that I would do the spotting of the pipe joint. I gave Jim compass commands, and he played the hydraulic levers like a concert pianist.

Since the ocean's sand floor was higher than the bottom of the pipeline, we had to jet down each section — a simple task — using a force-canceling nozzle designed for jetting and containing holes that directed half the force backwards. This enabled the diver to control it rather than the water's jetting forces controlling the diver. Once the pipe was jetted clear, I had Jim lower it until the flanges were aligned. I inserted a single bolt at three o'clock to secure the pipe ends together, then set in the large gasket and added three more bolts. After I had all four bolts tight, I came up and Hughie went down to install the rest and tighten them up. When he arrived back on deck, I went down and checked the torque of each bolt before moving the spar buoys for the next joint. My last task was to release the horse and come up. We averaged one-and-a-half joints a day and, in spite of our new foreman's inexperience, the job went surprisingly well.

While I was on the bottom, perhaps a week into the job, Woody's compressor threw a rod and left a large hole in the engine block. I came up cursing Mr. Treen and his number-one man, Willie. We were in a pickle. It was noon and our shift could not end until we released the pipe from the horse which were both still on the ocean floor. The only other compressor on board was a very large rotary unit which was used for airlifts and pile-driving hammers. It emitted a large volume of oil — not a healthy situation for breathing air.

Verne and Pierre volunteered to make a massive filter manifold of six two-feet high, four-inch steel pipes welded to the deck, and we filled them with Kotex to absorb the oil. I went ashore to purchase the Kotex. A lot of it.

("Yes ma'am," I told the salesperson, "six boxes of your super size. It's my wife's time and she's a big gal." The girl at the counter appeared perplexed; she probably wondered if my wife was the largest woman in Eureka. Though the town was home to some of the very hefty ladies who ran with the loggers, none probably ever ordered six boxes of super size at one time!)

Pierre tightened the last pipe cap onto the manifold, and Hughie went down to release the pipe from the horse. On the bottom, the always-gentle demeanor of my diving partner suddenly changed as he began voicing a stream of very harsh curses. Suspecting a judgment-altering buildup of carbon monoxide, I ordered Verne to bring him up.

Back on deck, though Hughie's normal personality returned, his ability to breathe did not. His lungs had been temporarily filled with oil and carbon monoxide and he was gasping for air. We administered oxygen from our cutting torch which relieved my diving partner's problem but left him very weak. I volunteered to go down and, though I suffered the same consequences, I managed to release the horse.

When I was back on deck, I lay over a deck box gasping, breastplate and all. Verne handed me the open oxygen torch hose and I cupped it over my face, breathing deeply. I was soon able to sit and be dressed out, seemingly none the worse for the experience. (I ended up fighting oil in my lungs for years, however, while Hughie suffered no long-term effects. This complicated my arguments with Mr. Treen who later refused to discuss the episode with me.)

I called Woody that night to have Willie bring up a new compressor. "What the hell do you mean, the compressor threw a rod?!" he yelled. "It must have been something you did. Our equipment is always in the best repair. In any case, we don't have another. You'll have to find one in Eureka." When I attempted to tell him about the oil in my lungs, Woody hung up.

Paving compressors should not be used for diving because their engine oil system is common to the compressor. The one I found, however, worked very well, delivering better air than Woody's green machine had delivered before it expired. Our jobs were saved, at least for the moment, and we went back to laying pipe. The Kotex-filled pipes ended up in the junk pile where Woody's compressor should have been in the first place.

With the exception of the never-ending high seas, our task continued smoothly for several more joints. Then we realized we had a serious problem. Because the grade of the ocean's floor was more level than that of our declining pipeline's slope angle, each joint had to be jetted further down than the last in order to align the flanges. I did my best to explain this to our foreman and, when Delbert had a difficult time comprehending our situation, several of the crew illustrated it on deck using soapstone and rather strong lingo.

I asked to have the horse lowered over the last joint we had made up. My plan was to jet two slings under it, make them up, and slowly milk the pipeline up by careful extensions of the horse's legs. As Jim brought up pressure, I would go along with the jet and free the pipe, breaking suction under it. I estimated it would take three hours to accomplish this.

"Oh bull," Del responded. "That will take too long. I'll have the boys rig up a twelve-by-twelve timber with weights so it will slightly sink. You rig a sling around the last flange, and I'll have Hank take a strain with the crane. When the pipe is up and free of the bottom, slip the timber under its end."

"Good grief, Del," I said, my face now beet red, "the tip of the crane's boom is going up and down ten feet. We'll break the pipe and end up in real trouble, beside's killing me in the process."

Delbert had his way and did indeed come close to killing me. Looking back, when I was overruled I should have asked to go in on the tug; a quitter, but an alive one.

I was not the only unhappy camper, for the entire crew thought Del's solution was crazy. Hank and I were both hyper-ventilating, and he was considering taking the tug ashore as well. We should have tossed Del overboard without a life vest, for the little bastard deserved it.

Standing on the twelve-by-twelve to position it, I put the sling around the end of the last pipe flange and I put its bitter end into the crane's hook. When the pipe end came up, I was to slide the timber under it with my foot; another game of Russian roulette, this time with a fifteen-thousand-pound guillotine. All in the dark.

My tender Pierre told me the load was coming up. My hand was on the pipe's offshore flange, touch being the only way I could tell if it was moving. It had not budged. I asked Pierre to confirm his previous statement and he did. Suddenly the pipe leaped up, as free of my touch as a soldier fleeing a foxhole. I had no idea where or how high the end of the pipe went or where I was. I was being flushed down a massive toilet alongside a fifteen-ton roller that the devil himself was swinging in an attempt to crush the very life from me and my new helmet.

Then I heard a dull, heavy thud. The pipe had somehow landed on the bottom without mashing me. But before I could rejoice, the entire sequence was repeated as the tip of the barge's boom once again raised up to the heavens, tossing the pipe about like a cat with a mouse.

This time the whirling waters and intense suction pulled me close to the surface. I could tell where I was because the coffee-colored water had lightened up. I was here, there, upside down, rightside up — an olive in a blender, doing my best to clear my ears and prevent the blowing out of my eardrums.

"Have Hank set the damned pipe on the bottom!" I screamed to Pierre. My tender had already given these orders, bypassing our chisel-nosed foreman who still had no idea what was taking place. Even before Pierre gave the order, Hank had taken the same liberty with the words, "All off. The pipe is on the bottom. I hope to God Kirby isn't under it." He later told me that he spoke these words with trembling hands and tear-filled eyes.

I regained my composure, located the end of the pipe, and began searching for the weighted timber. After a lengthy period of time, I found it ten feet on the other side. I could just as easily have ended up in the same place, only I would have been in far worse condition, following the journey, than the timber.

It is my guess that God decided to forgive me for my evil ways as a youth. From that moment on, I became a Believer. And I have not changed my view since.

Del's squeaky voice came over my phones. "Is the pipe okay?" he asked.

"How the hell would I know," I answered. "I need to take a look. It's my guess, however, that the pipe is broken." I slid my hands down the first joint and onto the second. These pipes were secure. I had soon inspected three joints and all were in good order. Just beyond the flange of the third joint, however, was a clean break. In order to repair the line, we would have to undo all four joints and set them on deck. I didn't say a word about this; I simply informed Pierre I was coming up.

My helmet was removed. Standing in front of me, his white hard hat low over his beady eyes, was Delbert De Witt. "How is the pipe?" he asked. Verne placed his hand on my shoulder and gave me a squeeze of understanding as he handed me a cup of coffee.

"Del," I answered, "the frigging fourth joint broke just like I said it would. We will now have to set the horse and begin to unbolt each joint. All because you are a pigheaded dick from the sticks. You came close to killing me..." I continued my tirade, loosing a string of colorful adjectives that described the miserable little foreman. I have never been known to stutter.

We set the horse over the last joint, I jetted slings under it and unbolted its flange, and Jim came up on the horse until they were tight, and that joint of pipe was then lifted onto the deck. By the end of our shift, two of the four joints were sitting alongside one another – not bad for an afternoon's effort.

It was then time to go in for the weekend. The barge was backed off, all anchor lines were slackened, and Del suggested I load my personal belongings onto the tug. I knew why.

Every Friday, Hughie and I would visit the hospital, give Norm a rundown on what had been accomplished that week, and he would hand us our checks. This time I was instructed to visit Norm by myself. Del De Witt was standing next to Norm's bed; he held his white hard hat in trembling hands. Norm handed me my check, then began with a very short, but to the point, tongue lashing.

"You broke my pipe," he said. "You're fired."

As the old saying goes, "Crap runs downhill." Norm and Del obviously needed a fall guy. Norm had already called Healy Tibbett's home office telling them someone had broken the pipe, Norm had protected Del.   My ability as a quality diver, our accomplishments, or the pain and risks we had encountered were of no importance. I was simply the person in line for the fall. It was a tough pill to swallow, of course, for I was fired after doing an outstanding job.

The next day as I headed south through the redwoods with my family, I assumed I was leaving company politics and the project behind. However, this was not the case. When I stepped into Woody's office the following day, he turned in his overstuffed leather chair while pointing a finger at me. "Kirby," he announced, "You broke the damned pipe. You're fired."

I did my best to befriend and assist Woody over the ensuing years but, one way or another, I always seemed to end up as the bad guy or I ended up on the short end of the rope. Still, we enjoyed many good times together. Though I prefer to remember these good times, they never made up for the bad ones. When I think of my experience with Healy Tibbetts Construction Company, I wonder why Woody didn't attempt to locate a diving compressor. Apparently, he just didn't care.

I never ran again ran into Norm or Del — a double blessing.

In October, 1998, I received word that Woody had passed on to the big decompression chamber in the sky. The short man with brown wavy hair and flamboyant personality was gone. This I did not wish to hear. In spite of the past with its occasionally painful memories, I loved Woody. Everyone did.

Winners And Losers

There are three kinds of people, I've heard it said
There are winners and losers and those who are dead
The dead do not count and the losers are tragic

But the winners are gifted with some kind of magic
You can't call it luck because luck is too fickle
One man's cucumber is another man's pickle

The noisy complainers harangue and harass
While the quiet achiever sits first in his class
Some have it easy and some have it tough

But the stayers comes through when the going gets rough
Stubborness wins though the vision be narrow
The way of the bow is the way of the arrow

G.G. Ainsworth

THE KIRBY MORGAN CORPORATION

Returning from my near-death experience, I gave Bev a rundown. After a few chuckles accompanied by raised eyebrows, we went over the many advances Bev had made during my absence. I was impressed. I returned to my work bench, making diving equipment. Reluctantly, I sold Orville to Woody. With the exception of teaching diving in college and occasionally getting wet, I would never again accept another commercial diving job.

Our abalone mask had evolved into a design incorporating a demand regulator using a port retainer that was upturned at the bottom to give the regulator clearance. The mask had a glued-in face seal, one earphone and, all in all, was a very pleasing unit. However, it had two outstanding drawbacks; it was almost impossible to clear our ears, and the regulator became very hard breathing at any depth beyond twenty feet.

Pete Brumis suggested using our plunging nose-clearing device, a simple invention that has lasted the test of time and is still being used by Diving Systems today.

Solving the problem of breathing resistance at depth was more involved. I had run into the same situation on the second mask I built on the naval ship during my 1955 abalone days. Because there were no single hose units on the market, this metal mask also incorporated a demand regulator that I had to design and fabricate. The thing worked well on deck and in shallow water, but at sixty feet it was almost impossible to get air. More on this, but first I need to explain the reasons for using a demand regulator in favor of the standard steady-flow air systems.

To begin with, I could use a smaller compressor. If the compressor should fail, and it often did, my volume tank would sustain adequate breathing air for a considerable time; this was not the case when using a free-flow mask that used three or four times the volume of air.

In addition, a reduction of exhaust bubbles took place when using a demand system. The exhaust from free-flow masks causes a constant head shaking which can be very tiring. The racket from the bubbles exiting a free-flow mask also makes it difficult for the diver to hear the tender's voice. This same exhaust garbling is picked up by the diver's earphones, hindering his voice transmissions to the surface.

Note: Effective communications with topside is the dividing line between commercial and sport diving. (Safe) commercial construction diving cannot take place unless there is a viable system of audible communications between the diver and topside.

I designed my San Diego abalone mask's regulator to operate on the surface, using about eighty pounds of supply pressure. Since it had a downstream inlet valve, a spring was necessary to hold back the air pressure on deck. When using surface-supplied air — at sixty feet of depth for instance — the effective air pressure was only fifty-three pounds instead of its original eighty on deck. The end result was that the closing spring's tension was then far too strong, hindering my inhalation effort — perhaps preventing it altogether.

> Note: Bev Morgan and Pat Kern did not run into this problem when they designed Wilson's system because their gas supply was mounted on the bell, and at roughly the same depth as the diver.

I overcame this problem by soldering a brass water valve into the side of my regulator, which was in alignment with the downstream valve's closing spring and inlet valve. This allowed me to adjust the closing spring's tension under water. My invention, which eventually became known as "Dial-a-Breath," worked very well. One year later, I allowed a Morro Bay abalone diver to talk me out of my mask with the experimental regulator. What a blunder.

Bev and I hired Agonic Machine Shop to machine this same adjustment system for our newly chosen demand regulator, the U.S. Divers Conshelf XII. It worked like a dream, and its basic theme is still used on many of the present masks and helmets produced by Diving Systems International (now named Kirby Morgan Dive Systems).

Agonic Machine later decided to form a new manufacturing company which they named General Aquadyne. They used our adjustable demand system to penetrate commercial diving equipment sales. Soon after, Scubapro snatched the invention and, for years, used it on many of their scuba regulators. I often wish I had patented the design, but I didn't have the necessary bucks. Besides, my crystal ball was full of kelp.

We continued to improve our devices on a daily basis. We would build and sell two or three masks in order to secure funding for our next design. During this approximately two-year period, our shop was essentially an R and D facility, not a production house. It would remain so until we developed a mask with a removable face seal and hood; a design that was decent enough to commit to a long production run.

During the years 1965 and '66, we also built an improved heavy gear air hat. We considered this helmet to be the ultimate in heavy gear, offering its basic frame as a recirculator. This design became known as the Kirby Morgan Commercial Helmet which is still prized by its owners today.

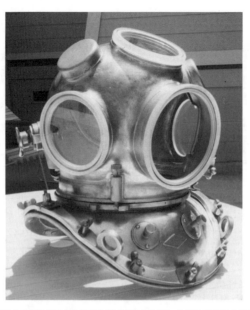

KIRBY MORGAN COMMERCIAL AIR HELMET #1

During 1966, Meribeth Treen, Woody's wife, made a trip to Japan where she visited with Mr. Tanaka, manager of Yokohama Diving Apparatus Company. Noticing one of our recirculators sitting on the floor (the one that had been ordered by Del Thomason) she asked Mr. Tanaka, "What is one of Bob Kirby's helmets doing here?"

"Oh no, Mrs. Treen," he said, "Dan Wilson designed that helmet. We are in the process of manufacturing it for him."

Meribeth convinced Mr. Tanaka that Bev Morgan and I had built that helmet, and he wrote us a letter of apology, promising never again to make a recirculator using our design.

Bev and I talked it over. We had not sold a recirculator or a commercial heavy gear hat in some time. We wrote Mr. Tanaka and gave him permission to continue making and selling our helmets plus the new and improved air hat we sent him — with no royalties to be paid. We felt honored to be in a position to assist such a fine, old firm. Should we receive requests for either style helmet in the future, we could order them from Yokohama Diving Apparatus and re-sell them to our customers.

Years later, following the death of Mr. Tanaka, Yokohama Diving Apparatus failed. I have no idea what happened to the company's inventory or tooling, but I would love to have it today.

At the end of 1965, we left the one-room building next to Associated Divers in Goleta and moved fifty yards north, into the old two-story stucco airline terminal. It was in poor condition, and we set about cleaning it up while moving in our equipment and belongings. Bev owned a large and very heavy oak desk that he had restored and refinished himself — a desk he was very proud of. It needed to be placed upstairs, a daunting task to say the least. The truck crane from my pile-driving days was parked outside, and I talked Bev into letting me lift his desk to the second-story veranda. We could then slide it through the large door overlooking the airport. Bev rigged his masterpiece, securing it for a safe and slow vertical lift.

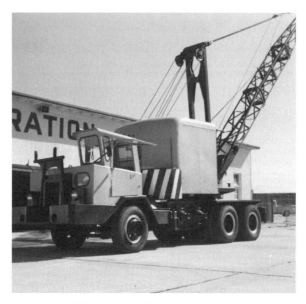

KIRBY TRUCK CRANE, 1966

This was not what I had in mind, however. Once the desk was high enough to clear the buildings, I began to swing it in a giant circle, intending to scare the crap out of my new partner. I succeeded in upsetting him, alright. The slings came loose, and his prize ended up barely hanging by one leg. Bev was furious at me for the rest of the day; hell, he was angry for a week, and he certainly let me know it. I often reflect on this, wondering what would have happened to our partnership if his desk had crashed to the ground. I was once again reminded that, perhaps, God really loved me.

The only other time I was the recipient of negative attention from Bev was in 1966 or '67, when I was to test a swim helmet recirculator we had built for the navy. We had installed a two-story water tank for testing gear at the side of our building. A square window at the bottom of the tank allowed us to observe the diver – when the water was clear, that is. On the day I was to test the navy's recirculator, the water was rusty as hell; a brown soup containing chunks of crud and resembling water in a sewer filtration plant.

The entrance to the tank was at the top of the same stairs that opened onto our building's second story and, for a reason I will never know, once I was dressed in I did a cannonball into the tank. I then waited on the bottom, in front of the viewing window, for my partner to arrive. When he didn't show, I called to him over our speaker system. "Hey, Bev! It's me, Bob. I'm on the bottom, waiting for you. Bev. Where are you? I'm still here."

After a long pause I heard his voice. "Come up, damn it!"

I had no idea why he wanted to terminate the dive, for everything was working as planned. "Bev," I said, "I'm on the bottom. I need you."

"Goddamn it!" Bev yelled. "Come up!"

My partner seldom swore so, up I came. It didn't take long to understand his unusual demeanor. My acrobatics had flooded the upstairs room with perhaps fifty gallons of rusty brown tank water which was running down our newly painted lower walls and over Bev's many prized photos; photos which Bev had taken himself, then had carefully framed and hung. A skilled cameraman, Bev was very proud of these photographs. He was sensitive about their being touched by human hands, let alone by an onslaught of rusty water. The wonderful photos were now buckling up like wrinkled skin, and I spent the rest of the day cleaning while Bev attempted to restore his artwork. He still recalls this event with anger; and it's no wonder he fired me in 1980. If I had been in his shoes, I would have been fired much sooner.

I had invented the adjustable demand regulator and many of the Kirby recirculator heavy gear hats. My understanding of demand regulators, my mechanical knowledge, and my metal-working skills were indisputable. Bev had his own share of inventions, however, inventions that were equal to and, in many ways, surpassed mine. He had spent far more hours than I as an abalone diver and, because he had used swim gear exclusively, he was able to exploit his broad knowledge concerning its good and bad points. His talent and understanding of human factors was incredible. By combining my mechanical design work and abilities using metal with Bev's many talents, a dynamic team was created that has not been equaled since.

When we added the adjustable demand system, our new mask line was looking very good. The design still needed one major improvement, however, and this would be Bev's invention − the mask's removable hood and improved face seal. This invention would take place in the future; for the time being, we lived with the glued-in face seals which were far better than any other commercial diving masks on the market.

Suddenly, for some reason we did not understand, our sales began to drop, and I was assigned to fly to the gulf and do my best to sell our new mask line. I had no idea what to expect in Louisiana. When I arrived, I found many divers were still using the old Jack Browne mask, a Desco design that was created during the WWII. Since these masks came minus communications, some of the companies using them had installed a single large speaker in the view port, thus obstructing the already limited visibility. The diver was forced to shout his words; then,in order to hear the reply he would turn off his air. This system was but one step better than two tin cans connected by a tight string.

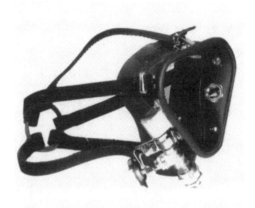

JACK BROWNE MASK

Once I had penetrated the southern accents — a tough call in itself — I realized the two Cajuns running their diving firm were struggling to explain that they did not <u>want</u> communications with topside. This, after I had pointed out that the ability to converse would speed up the dive.

One looked at me in amazement. "Why de hell y'all want speed up de job? We get pay by de shift. Yo' new mask gone cause us *no money*. Y'all *stupid* or somethin'?"

By the end of the week, after accruing no sales, I drove west to World Wide Divers in Morgan City, Louisiana. Ex-divers Johnny Johnson and Mike Hughes owned this firm and are friends today. Though they understood my logic, they ordered only two masks, for they had plans involving Bob Ratcliff who was working on a new helmet in back of their shop, a design that eventually became the famous "Rat hat."

Shortly after my trip to Louisiana, World Wide merged with Can Dive and Cal Dive to form Oceaneering, and they planned to use Bob Ratcliff's Rat Hat exclusively. Years later, Oceaneering grew so rapidly that they ended up buying our equipment as well.

Bob Ratcliff was another of the pioneers at General Offshore Diving during the heydays of Dan Wilson and the *Purisima* bell system. On my trip to World Wide, Bob proudly displayed his new design, a very original dry swim helmet.

I finished my trip with a visit to J and J Divers in Houston, owned by John Galletti and Joe Carroll. John and Joe, like John and Mike at World Wide, had started out as diving partners and had gone on to build a highly successful diving service. Two years earlier, before I went into partnership with Bev Morgan, Joe Carroll had arrived at my shop next to Associated Divers, and he had purchased one recirculator heavy gear helmet. Both Joe and John were delighted by my visit, and they ordered four masks. This purchase accelerated our trend. We were on our way. Had it not been for their orders, I expect our fledgling firm would have perished.

We now had enough work to continue until orders started coming in over the phone again. Lee Hixon, owner of a diving company in Santa Monica, ordered a mask and, though he had a reputation for not paying his bills, we shipped him a mask of our latest design. The mask cost $600, but Lee never paid. He called, begging Bev to send him a second mask. Bev appeared very sympathetic. "Lee wants another mask. I told him I'd send him one, and I will."

Bev packed up a couple quarts of resin, some paint brushes, glass cloth, and sandpaper (enough items to equal the weight of a mask) and placed it in one of our shipping boxes. Bev included in the box a slip of paper reading, "Diving Mask Kit," and he shipped it for $600, C.O.D.

Several months later, Lee called again. This time he needed a recirculator helmet, and my partner agreed to order one from Yokohama Diving Apparatus, contingent upon Lee picking it up himself (along with some other conditions). Lee was to pay us $1300 in one-dollar bills, and the money was to be delivered by a card-carrying prostitute who would perform any act requested by anyone in the building. Lee agreed to this.

Two months later Lee drove in; sitting alongside Lee was a redhead with large jugs. She was slightly over the hill, but still very attractive. Lee carried a large sack into the shop and dumped 1300 one-dollar bills on the floor, creating quite a mound of money. The redhead followed him and, after looking around, eventually rested her eyes on Bev who was wearing a subdued smile.

Hixon spoke up. "Guys, I want you to meet my wife. She won't go along with your crap."

In addition to the normal face seal, our mask had a hood glued in. This design accommodated the two earphones, and a zipper down the back enabled the unit to dry out. It worked, but the face seal was uncomfortable on long dives, and gluing them in place was a pain. One day in or around 1967, Bev came up with the answer; a hood with the face seal attached to it, not to the mask frame. This one-piece rubber unit was then clamped onto the body of the mask. Its best feature was a stretched-across face seal that was far more comfortable than the glued-in original — a stroke of genius that was as good as anything I had ever come up with.

Bev then went to work on the tough job of redesigning the frame to clear the diver's chin, while I designed and made the band holding the hood/face seal assembly to the frame. The "Band Mask" was born.

If there is such a thing as a "bumper year," the year 1967 was to be ours. The mask was well-thought-out and became the first of our assembly line. However, neither of us enjoyed production and, since we couldn't afford to hire a man to do the dirty work, I tolerated it by placing myself in a trance and playing games to increase production, while Bev grumbled and made excuses in order to avoid the hours of sticky resin and itchy cloth. I couldn't blame him.

During this production, with its ensuing drudgery, our main entertainment was a new swim helmet design that we had started to work on after I returned from the gulf. Ours was a totally different design from the Rat Hat designed by Bob Ratcliff. Calling it the SemiLite, it used the same mask front as that on our band mask while blending in and becoming a fiberglass shell all the way. We encountered a host of problems; some were never resolved, spelling a short life for our flamboyant masterpiece. However, we learned several things that became stepping stones for our future helmet, the SuperLite 17. The SuperLite 17 was to become the "Model A Ford" of the diving helmet industry, a wonderful helmet that was in production for over a quarter of a century. (This effort, however, would wait until 1975.)

In-water testing was essential, for one dive is worth a train-full of theories. We had yet to build another test tank, so we sweet-talked the owners of a neighboring motel into occasionally renting us their pool. This was not so easy, for we were never able to make good our promise to install a water dust trap that would keep our fiberglass grindings from contaminating their downwind facilities. The owners grumbled about our presence in the pool while their patrons enjoyed the entertainment. The patrons, mainly women, would stand on the upper veranda, support their breasts on the hand rail, and gaze at history being made by two madmen covered with fiberglass dust − as was the motel.

I had no appreciation of how much ballast would be needed by the SemiLite hats, or where the ballast should be placed. I ended up casting pockets of lead inside, a very poor idea as this is where our heads belonged. To achieve watertight integrity, we had a wet suit neck dam pulled tight around the helmet's base. It was retained by a wire clamp. The diver had to stretch the neck opening to get his head through; an effort suggesting a trip back into the womb.

The design had a face seal within. A rubber strap grabbed the lower back of the diver's head, just below his skull, pulling his face into the seal. This strong strap also cut off circulation and resulted in a migraine headache.

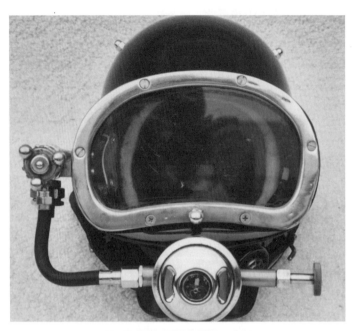
SEMILITE HELMET, 1966

It was one thing to test the helmet in a swimming pool and quite another to try it out in God's ocean using a scuba bottle. Bev warned me this was a stupid idea. Should I run out of air and have to ditch out, I would either lose the hat or be forced to swim with twenty-seven pounds of helmet in my arms. Buoyancy compensators had not yet been invented. But, without letting Bev know, I went ahead with my crazy scheme. No one could tell me anything, for I considered myself to be the world's best diver. Considering the many mishaps I had encountered over the years, one would think I would have learned something. Instead, being a hopeless fool, I decided to take another risk.

I drove my family to San Simeon State Park, set up camp and, in the evening, enjoyed a cool drink and a hot meal. Claudia had no idea I might not be around for dinner the following evening. (Of course, neither did I.)

After breakfast we packed my equipment to the water's edge, and I assured my wife I knew exactly what I was doing. The ocean was placid and the water was as clear as it gets. The sand beach ran out at a very shallow angle and, after an underwater swim of twenty yards, I was in perhaps fifteen feet of water. Having a dry head was simply wonderful; I was warm as toast. The arrangement worked like a dream, and I was convinced Bev's concerns were groundless. What did he know, anyway? I was the trained navy diver, not him. Hadn't I received a written license to be in scuba gear after taking a brief scuba qualification course in the service? Screw Bev Morgan.

After fifteen minutes on the bottom, I was ready to return to shore, but I didn't have a compass. "Oh well," I told myself, "I'll just stick my head out of the water, look around, determine my location, and head for the beach."

This turned out to be an impossibility, for I could not swim hard enough to surface my view port. The helmet was too heavy. I had no idea what to do, short of ditching our prized hat. And if I didn't die during that undertaking, Bev would kill me when I arrived home minus our treasure. I was a dead man in either case.

We had put a lot of money into the hat's design, half his and half mine. Still, I was about to abandon every penny when I noticed small sand riffles on the bottom, parallel to the shoreline. Heading one direction would take me out to sea, the other direction led to safety. Taking my best shot, I swam against the direction of the riffles. It worked, and I emerged from the water, shaken but safe. When I told Bev about the incident later, he used the same adjectives he had used when I almost dropped his desk onto the tarmac.

Band Mask sales soared. Coming up with names for all our different models was tough because we made so many changes along the way. We named our latest model the KMB (Kirby Morgan Band Mask) 8, and counted backwards to the KMB 6. We did not assign names to earlier models as they had very limited production runs; sometimes only one or two.

It became apparent we were under-funded and, in order to increase production, we needed outside money so that we could hire a necessary troop or two. We began looking around for someone to invest in our fledgling firm. Bob Christensen, an old friend of ours, said he had heard that a Santa Barbara corporation, Pacific Instruments, wanted to get involved in undersea activity, and a meeting was arranged. Looking back, that meeting was a dismal day in our lives, if not in the history of diving. As I've often said before, crap happens. This time there would be enough crap to fill our two-story test tank.

PACIFIC INSTRUMENTS INCORPORATED

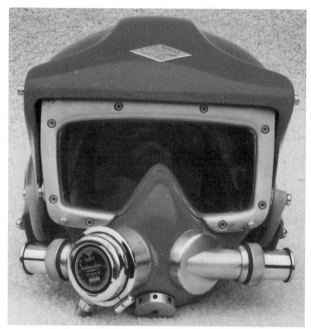 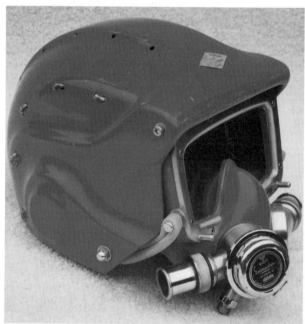

CLAMSHELL HELMET

The crap arriving in 1968 was delivered in a large drum labeled "Lots of Crap," and it began to leak all over the place.

Bev and I were unable to maintain production of diving masks while continuing to work on the Navy's Sea Lab Clamshell helmets, a contract we had just been awarded to produce over a dozen special hats. In retrospect, we should have toughed it out; instead, we decided to expand, and for this we needed a money transfusion in order to hire help and enlarge our operation. As I mentioned earlier, Bob Christensen, an old friend who had been both a military diver and a commercial diver, suggested we talk to Pacific Instruments, a Santa Barbara Corporation involved in the electronics manufacturing business that had expressed an interest in our fledgling underwater industry. Bob set up a meeting with their vice president, Harry Appleborne, for us to discuss a merger. The fact that this appointment turned out to be a black day in our lives is no reflection on Harry, for he was a prince, but he did not understand our market or how to handle commercial divers. He also had no idea that the Richard Regan, president of Pacific Instruments hoped to eliminate Harry.

Our cold offshore world of heavy construction, rusty boats, and hard-drinking fast-fisted honest roughnecks was not the same world inhabited by those in the instrument manufacturing field. That world was inhabited by troops of exacting workers who were glued to clean, white Formica, fluorescent-lit workbenches. The attempt to merge individuals from two worlds with such fundamentally incompatible philosophies was doomed from the beginning.

Even worse, Harry maintained a foolish faith in Regan, a supposedly close friend with whom he had founded the firm. Regan, in his stylish suit and sporting a broad smile, was a salesman who felt no remorse when screwing others. Including his partner, Harry Appleborne.

Harry proceeded to formulate the merger of Kirby Morgan Corporation with Pacific Instruments. Bev and I would each receive ten percent of the business as would Harry; Pacific would pick up the balance of the stock and pledge a $20,000 line of credit at the bank. Should we need more than twenty grand, we would fall back and regroup. Neither Harry, Bev, nor I had any idea that this last statement meant the end of the Kirby Morgan Corporation unless we could buy our way out of bondage — a tough call at that time.

The merger was part of Regan's plan to rid himself of Harry, for he planned to force us into bankruptcy. It appears that though Regan had tolerated Appleborne for years, they mixed like water and oil. Harry rubbed against Regan at every turn; both of their bodies were covered with sores. It was amazing that Harry did not have a clue as to Regan's plan to shame him into retiring. Bev and I didn't see it coming either. We figured both of them were good guys.

Once the paperwork had been completed, new tools began to show up — Harry's acquisitions — and I thanked God for this blessing because most of our tools were pieces of rust with broken handles. My hand tools were so old they looked as if they had come around the horn on a sailing ship, and I had purchased most of my electric tools from Clark's Used Tool Exchange on lower State Street. They looked that way — used.

With the exception of his paint brushes hanging by their handles in a covered bucket of diesel oil, Bev's tools looked even worse than mine. (Bev took great pride in his skill as a boat painter and, reflecting this pride, his paint bristles were fine and straight. He had no patience with sloppy work, especially in the painting department.)

Harry's second acquisition was a helper to assist in laying up fiberglass. This young man, Skip Dunham, continued with Bev and, around 1975, became president of Diving Systems International. However, when we hired him he needed training...a lot of it.

Skip's first task was to assist in painting the shop's interior, for the walls still showed evidence of its earlier dousing with rusty water. As I mentioned, the desk incident, my cannonball into the swimming pool, and Bev's encounter with Walt Swenson were three times I had seen my partner mad. He was angered a fourth time when Skip, doing his best as a painter, not only destroyed one of Bev's fine paint brushes but also ended up with as much paint on himself as on the wall. Bev walked in to find our new employee, hands covered with wet paint, holding onto a newly covered work bench while attempting to drink coffee from a slippery, paint-covered cup.

"Get the hell out!" Bev yelled. "And don't come back until I call you!" Skip, his hands still sticky with wet paint, got in his car and drove off.

Two days later, Bev phoned Skip. "Okay, dammit, you can come back. But you had better clean up your act." Bev, who had calmed down, was in charge, or so he thought. But, in fact, it was Harry who was now in charge, for Pacific Instruments Incorporated now owned over half our operation.

I began noticing a change in Bev's demeanor when Harry announced we would be dropping the Bank Mask line as well as all our other diving equipment. Both Bev and I were confused by this as we had a contract with the navy for the Clamshell helmets, and this was a task we had to complete or we might be looking at reams of legal documents from Uncle Sam.

Nevertheless, Harry had determined we could not make adequate money manufacturing diving masks or doing anymore work for the navy. Of course, as we later realized, the actual culprit was Dick Regan who was poking Harry with a sharp stick at every opportunity.

In the electronic industry, items are marketed at five times the actual cost for materials and labor. In Bev and my world, twice-direct costs were the best we could do; leaving us enough money, perhaps, to cover our still reasonably small overhead. For instance, we rented the two-story 1930 airline terminal for $125 a month. When Harry hired a secretary and ordered us to refuse any further mask sales, we began to get poorer day by day. Then he announced we were going into the underwater light business.

Bev drifted further and further from our assigned tasks and would just sit at his desk and sulk. But I really liked Harry and I wanted our firm to succeed, even if we were only manufacturing underwater lights.

However, we never got the chance. One day Dick Regan showed up with his arms filled with papers. "Okay guys," he announced. "It's all over. You have exceeded Pacific's pledge. You are now broke. I suggest you lock the doors and go home. There will be no further pay checks."

I sat, coffee cup in hand, on the second-floor veranda with Bev, and we discussed the situation. Five months earlier my friend and partner and I had been in the black; barely, but still, we had been there. Now we owed $20,000 and possessed only a handful of new tools to show for it. Not only that, but we had turned down all customers who called wanting diving masks. As far as the diving industry was concerned, we were history. Even worse, we had to continue with the navy's order for Clamshell hats or hire a lawyer, for we had no idea how to get out of that can of worms.

Bev met with Pete Brumis who agreed to lend Bev the $20,000. We could pay back Pacific and be independent again. I was invited to share in the note but declined. I had no idea where the bucks would come from if I was to continue. I had no idea if my decision to leave was good or bad. I will never know.

While sitting on the veranda with Bev, pondering my next move, my senses had been sharpened. Once again I was captured by the smell of aviation gasoline and the thunder of the huge radial engines. Now free, I would choose aviation as my next field. Even though I stayed with it only six years, this was a choice I never regretted, for those were some of the most exciting years of my life — second only to diving. For six winters and summers we built them, flew them, and wrecked them. God but it was fun!

I flew airliners filled with tons of oil drilling equipment over the Brooks Range in Alaska — this was like driving huge trucks that could fly. I ended up in fights, rolling in the snow with dirty-necked ruffnecks, and I held my own at the bargaining table as well. Life was anything but dull, and the bottom line was this: I was very successful in the aviation business.

Dick Regan and his clean white rooms, lies, and miniskirted secretaries could go to hell. My scars from Pacific Instruments soon healed, and I was once again my own man. The pain of leaving my partner lingered, but I knew Bev and I would be together again one day.

Note: Bev and Skip completed the Clamshell helmet contract. In 1970 Bev sold the Band Mask line to U.S. Divers and, until 1974 when more ugliness raised its head, he enjoyed a decent lifestyle.

THE U.S. NAVY

This chapter is about our United States Navy; some of its diving history and our involvement with it. These are my views, seen through my eyes only. The chapter spans almost half-a-century. Good grief!

In order to keep dates and times intact, I shall have to skip around. Sorry about that. If you become concerned about times and places not agreeing, remember; this is not a stringent dissertation on diving history.

My involvement with the navy was a hit and miss adventure that took place over many years, beginning with my enlistment. As far as I know, Kirby Morgan is still doing business with our boys in blue.

During my enlistment as a navy diver, I never acquired a military frame of mind. In fact, the way Uncle Sam went about things upset me no end, and I often let my feelings be known. Other than upsetting others, then myself, and leaving a bitter taste in all our mouths, very little was ever accomplished. A third-class metal smith, second-class diver is as low as whale poop; a substance that lies on the ocean floor and has no clout whatsoever.

Eight years after I mustered out, I looked back on my military days with sadness. I then determined we could help the navy and perhaps even the score. Bev and I would attempt to construct better diving equipment for the navy, a simple solution.

I did not comprehend the magnitude of such an undertaking. In fact it took Bev over twenty years of endless efforts to make any significant progress. And, during my early attempts, I acquired few military friends while making many enemies. Trying to teach old chiefs new ways was as impossible as flying a cast-iron submarine over all of Europe.

Whenever I showed particular interest in a situation, Bev Morgan was there to support me. I felt the same about him. After some hesitation, though the navy had never entertained such an idea, Bev went along with my nutty plan to replace the navy's helium diving helmets with our more practical, civilian design. The navy, of course, didn't know anything about us; who we were or our reputation in the field of diving. Nor did they care.

When I was a second-class navy diver, qualifying on the ASR *Florican* and making our yearly deep descent to 150 feet in the Mark V equipment, the first-class divers were diving off the other side of the salvage tug using the same helmets, but theirs were fitted with helium recirculators which are all but impossible to use. Any leak was deadly. An hour could be spent painting the dressed-in diver with soapy water while checking for bubbles indicating leaks. I was sure the navy would love a better machine. I was dead wrong.

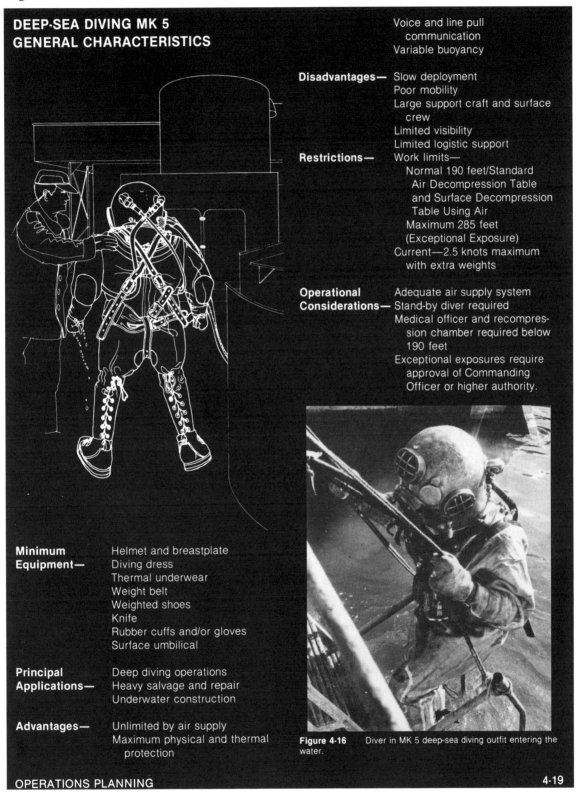

DEEP-SEA DIVING MK 5
GENERAL CHARACTERISTICS

	Voice and line pull communication
	Variable buoyancy
Disadvantages—	Slow deployment
	Poor mobility
	Large support craft and surface crew
	Limited visibility
	Limited logistic support
Restrictions—	Work limits—
	Normal 190 feet/Standard Air Decompression Table and Surface Decompression Table Using Air
	Maximum 285 feet (Exceptional Exposure)
	Current—2.5 knots maximum with extra weights
Operational Considerations—	Adequate air supply system
	Stand-by diver required
	Medical officer and recompression chamber required below 190 feet
	Exceptional exposures require approval of Commanding Officer or higher authority.

Minimum Equipment—	Helmet and breastplate
	Diving dress
	Thermal underwear
	Weight belt
	Weighted shoes
	Knife
	Rubber cuffs and/or gloves
	Surface umbilical
Principal Applications—	Deep diving operations
	Heavy salvage and repair
	Underwater construction
Advantages—	Unlimited by air supply
	Maximum physical and thermal protection

Figure 4-16 Diver in MK 5 deep-sea diving outfit entering the water.

In the latter half of 1965 I convinced Bev to allow me to rebuild a worn-out Mark V to our commercial recirculator configuration. We would then send it, gratis, to the Naval Experimental Unit, "EDU," in Washington, D.C. for evaluation. Even though we really couldn't afford this, we proceeded. We ended up with a beautiful (polished brass and all), modern rebuilt Mark V recirculator which was head and shoulders better than anything our navy had ever seen. We boxed it up, shipped it off, and expected instant feedback. It never materialized.

Instead, a couple months later, the battered crate was returned. The helmet and Sodasorb canister were intact and the brass components still shined. The converted Mark V had never seen the water.

Bev gave them a call. After some time he spoke to a commander who vaguely remembered the helmet, and the commander summoned the chief who had performed the evaluation. As it turned out, the helmet had been bounced about during shipment, and this had caused the Sodasorb to slightly powder. This is a common occurrence, and commercial divers dealt with it by ventilating each new load of absorbent before a dive. In the case of our Mark V, this seemingly obvious solution had been overlooked. Bottom line: the design was rejected because it presented a change.

I now had a couple thousand dollars of egg on my face. I salvaged the recirculator parts for use on a commercial hat and, after melting off the other components, I tossed the remainder of the Mark V in our scrap barrel. I wish I had it today, for it would not only be worth big bucks, but it would enjoy a place in diving history.

Looking back, it was probably a good thing the navy resisted our change because the saturation diving revolution all but retired our recirculators as well as theirs.

When young and energetic Commander John Harder took over EDU in 1967, he contacted Bev. A couple of small R and D projects were the result of this conversation; each project represented the magic number, $1000. A higher cost would have generated lots of paperwork.

The swim recirculator helmets that we were then tasked to construct cost us over $2000 to design and build, and we were foolish enough to believe there would be enough orders to put us ahead. Any decent businessman would have strung us up by our gonads.

The navy told us not to build the back pack recirculators as they would be using existing, well-tested, Mark VI units. Commander Harder could not loan us a Mark VI to test our helmets because his superior officers felt they had the market cornered on evaluation. We were requested to send completed, but untested, helmets; the navy would do all the testing.

Designing a mask attached to a swim helmet, one that could retain the recirculator's bag pressure, is somewhat dicey to begin with; not having a Mark VI to assist us, turned our

R and D efforts into an impossible situation. We were forced to make our own recirculator for testing the swim helmets; an expensive undertaking.

Our two wet helmet designs had been completed about a year apart and were plagued with problems. In order to overcome them, much research was required. We were never able to solve some of the problems, at least not to our satisfaction. It goes without saying that some of them would show up when designing future wet helmets.

Our method of designing was unorthodox, but it worked. We would try one thing, discard it, then try something else. Engineers in fluorescent-lit rooms would not have appreciated our hands-on approach, but their costly methods would have exceeded our $1000 contract several times over. We were small but efficient. When it came to the raw conceptual engineering of diving masks and helmets, no one could touch us.

In order to survive financially in those days, I spent a portion of each day laying up fiberglass for our production civilian masks. Bev did the same thing. While we were doing this we were also working out the design of fiberglass parts for our naval units and our new civilian units. We were as busy as could be and enjoying every minute of it; that is if hunger is ever enjoyable!

During that time we began to consider a new helmet and suit system designed to keep the diver dry while affording him the freedom of swimming. Bev, a commercial diver who had written a book or two and many magazine articles, devoted a dozen closely typed pages describing our concept, "DUDS" − Diver Underseas Diving System. This design was basically fiberglass heavy gear plus an ability to swim. The helmet would have a large rectangular view port and controls similar to those in our old abalone helmets.

At the time we thought this concept was greater than a bowl full of grits. In retrospect, it was one giant step backwards.

Before we could evaluate the new plan and determine its faults, my partner received a call from Captain Mickelson in Washington, D.C., Supervisor of Salvage. This man was no lightweight. He wanted to come out for a visit, and he would be armed with a briefcase filled with good news. The navy wanted to do business with us, and in a big way. We were beside ourselves with excitement. We were finally making a serious inroad into military diving. We would be rich and, for a change, our navy would be ending up with good gear.

The rental car pulled in alongside my truck crane and out stepped a tall, dapper man, finely appointed in his western outfit, hat and all. His bright shirt was adorned with all the trimmings, including a chrome-plated bolo tie depicting an Indian on a pony. The tips of his snakeskin boots were sharp enough to crush cockroaches caught in a corner, and the surface of his oval rhinestone belt buckle was large enough to contain a meal for an entire family.

Captain Mickelson removed his hat, revealing well-groomed, flowing gray hair. His eyes, a sparkling brown, were capped by sharp dark eyebrows. He was finely manicured and could have been a western movie actor.

"Okay guys," he said after relaxing in my chair and placing his snakeskin boots on my desk, "what do you have that is new?" (If he had confiscated Bev's chair and placed his boots on Bev's oak masterpiece, he would have found himself back in his rented Ford.)

Bev and I looked at one another. "Well," my partner began with hesitation, "we have a new design that is on paper only, and it allows a diver to stay warm and swim at the same time. I have it typed up, but we don't have the money to proceed with the hardware."

Bev sensed that our new acquaintance might be self-serving but, because we were committed, we had to play out our hand. Besides...perhaps, just perhaps...this guy might be genuine. Mickelson removed his boots from my desk, abandoned his "good old boy" demeanor and, acquiring a look of intention, began to read the twelve pages Bev had given him. He raised one eyebrow, then the other. The wheels were turning.

"Guys," he finally said, "this is great. I'll need a copy to take with me to D.C." Bev and I looked at one another; we had no other copy and copy machines had not yet been invented. After a long hesitation, we agreed to lend him the original to be copied and returned.

"What goes on in this town after dark?" was his next question. Though I knew what he was getting at, I decided to play dumb by inviting him to our home where he could bounce our son on his lap and enjoy a steak. The dapper captain did not answer; instead, he addressed Bev. Bev offered the same amenities, minus the baby bouncing.

"Oh no," the captain continued. "I mean what is taking place in the way of entertainment; you know...girls and things like that. The town; where's the action?" Saying little else, he swaggered to his car with our paperwork in his briefcase, and we never saw the paperwork or the captain again. Eight years later the navy came up with a design for a new helmet — the Mark XII. Its concept matched our DUDS plan exactly and was a disaster. We could have saved the navy a lot of trouble because, shortly after the captain departed, we scrapped the idea.

192

DEEP SEA DIVING MK 12
GENERAL CHARACTERISTICS

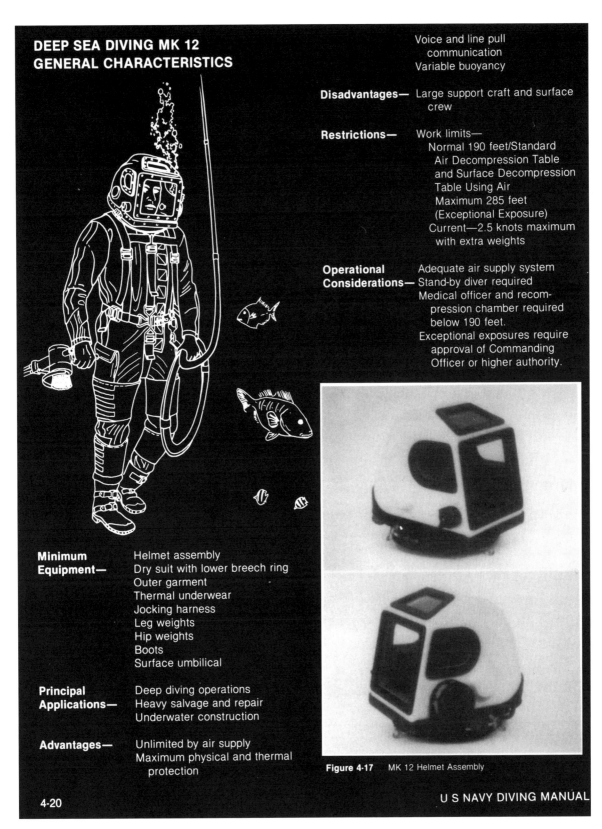

	Voice and line pull communication
	Variable buoyancy
Disadvantages—	Large support craft and surface crew
Restrictions—	Work limits— Normal 190 feet/Standard Air Decompression Table and Surface Decompression Table Using Air Maximum 285 feet (Exceptional Exposure) Current—2.5 knots maximum with extra weights
Operational Considerations—	Adequate air supply system Stand-by diver required Medical officer and recompression chamber required below 190 feet. Exceptional exposures require approval of Commanding Officer or higher authority.

Minimum Equipment—	Helmet assembly Dry suit with lower breech ring Outer garment Thermal underwear Jocking harness Leg weights Hip weights Boots Surface umbilical
Principal Applications—	Deep diving operations Heavy salvage and repair Underwater construction
Advantages—	Unlimited by air supply Maximum physical and thermal protection

Figure 4-17   MK 12 Helmet Assembly

4-20

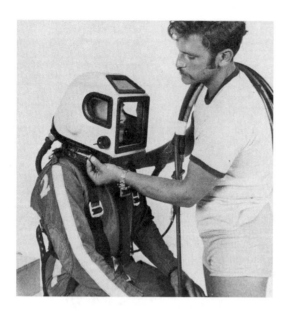

T Press the button on the quick-release locking pins and slide into place. Ensure that all pins are properly locked.

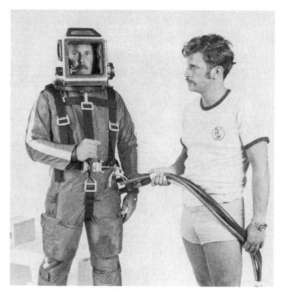

V The diver adjusts the front diving strap to his preference.

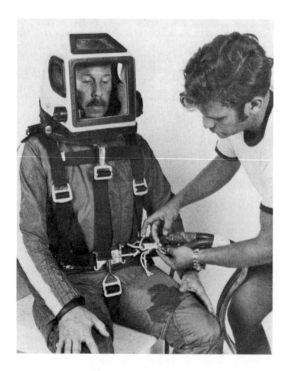

U Lead the umbilical and whips under the left arm to the wrist V-ring. Secure with the spinnaker-type snap shackle. Ensure that it is locked. Ensure that the quick-release cord is attached and in good condition.

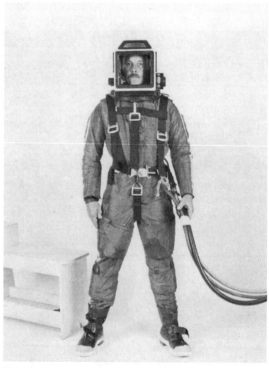

W With the diver fully dressed, perform a communications check (see MK 12 Operation and Maintenance Manual, NAVSEA 0994-LP-018-5010).

6-32

U S NAVY DIVING MANUAL

As previously related, I resigned from the Kirby Morgan Corporation in 1968. Then, in 1974, I rejoined Bev and we formed Diving Systems International. The catalyst for our new corporation was a helmet I had modified at home using the first yoke principal of retention. This little air helmet was a beauty, for it was comfortable and had excellent balance in the water. Bev and I were both in hog heaven, but we didn't have enough money to bring a new design to the market place. We needed to sell something in order to move ahead, and our new helmet was the only thing we could sell. Times were tough; nothing had changed.

The bamboo telegraph was working, and we soon got a call from Commander Barry Ridgewell, a Royal Canadian Navy exchange officer assigned to our navy's experimental diving unit, EDU, which had relocated in Panama City, Florida. Barry had been tasked to design and build the new USN Mark XII. This was outlined by a stack of papers, straight from the supervisor of salvage.

Ridgewell, a fine and intelligent man, recognized the shortcomings of the plastic heavy gear concept, and he wanted to move the project toward the direction Bev and I were now heading with our neutral buoyancy head-jocked swim hat.

Ridgewell made an appointment to visit us on the west coast and dive it at my home. He would be accompanied by five evaluation engineers. If they liked it, we might be able to work out a deal to make one for them.

By now we had gained experience working with civil engineers. As a rule, most of them didn't possess a sense of humor so, being somewhat evil, Bev and I came up with a plan. I purchased a regulation galvanized bucket at our local hardware store, and I soldered an old discarded Japanese view port onto its front. We glued foam inside the interior, so the thing could be suspended on the diver's head, and we attached a simple, stretched diaphragm of wet suit material under its rim.

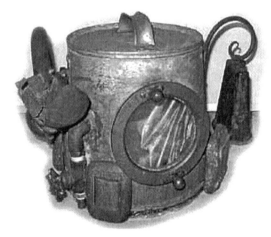

Bev Morgan
BUCKET HELMET

195

As our humorous design evolved, important features were added. A water valve was resurrected from my scrap pile to regulate the air supply, and on one side we attached an ornate brass hanger from which was suspended an old cowbell. The other side sported a bulb-style antique automobile horn. Then we attached a trunk handle to the top and snapped a scuba weight belt around the helmet's base. As a final touch, we proudly affixed our company name tag. To our amazement, the thing worked perfectly the first dive.

The day we were to unveil the world's newest and greatest swim helmet arrived. Two gray government vehicles showed up at my home by ten and Barry Ridgewell jumped out to greet us. The five engineers, all wearing inexpensive blue J.C. Penney suits, held back, eye-balling the swimming pool adjacent to our 1911 barn. They were obviously not too impressed by the pool, the two of us, or the old shed housing my blacksmith shop.

A blanket covered two lumps on a wooden table; one was the helmet we wanted to sell them and the other was the hat we had concocted with the bucket. As I slowly pulled back the blanket covering our galvanized monstrosity, the cowbell was the first thing they saw. Using a county fair, snake oil approach, I began my pitch. "This cowbell is for underwater communications. It works so well we intend to patent it. The auto horn will only work in the dry. It is to summon help when on the surface. The water valve is the best known. It can pass an adequate quantity of air and eliminates the harsh sound accompanying normal helmet valves. All in all, this helmet is a masterpiece. Bev and I are proud of it. We know you'll be eager to purchase it for five thousand bucks. You are getting a hell of a deal!"

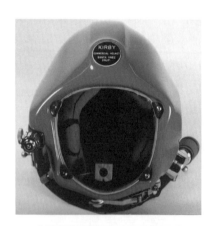

LITTLE RED HELMET

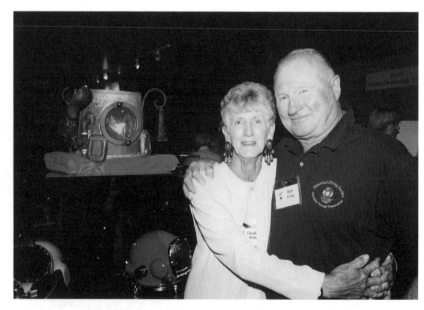

UNVEILING THE LITTLE RED HELMET

196

I finished my spiel and observed the five engineers returning to their cars. "Okay you two bastards," Ridgewell said with a grin. "Cut the crap. Where the hell is the real hat?"

I explained that messing with civil servants was my second hobby and that it took a back seat only to my self-appointed duty to upset fish and game wardens. When I removed the blanket and revealed our red prototype, the engineers returned.

Each engineer swam about in the pool, and they loved the swim hat. Then their attention was drawn to the bucket hat, and they spent a far longer time, clapping the bell and honking the horn, than they spent evaluating the real thing. The bucket hat won out and is held in high esteem at Diving Systems today, where it occupies the center position in their display case.

Barry Ridgewell wanted a helmet exactly like the one they had tested, but in blue instead of red. They would pay the agreed fee of $5000, and I winced and scratched my butt.

"Barry," I said, "that's a formidable job. I overheated the original mold and we'll have to make a new one."

This was entirely true, but what I didn't tell him was that we would be painting the red hat blue, and then sending it to them. Barry signed a purchase order, and a week later we shipped him the newly painted helmet. The money was ours.

Barry presented his new plan to his superiors, and they relayed it to the supervisor of salvage in Washington, D.C. In strongly enunciated wording, it was suggested he might find himself designing a lighthouse in Greenland if he continued to deviate from his original orders. The Mark XII was to be built to the specifications depicted on the stack of paper work on his desk. There would be no room for games. He was to no longer entertain a head-mounted swim helmet, and he was to destroy our purchase order and forget Bev Morgan and Bob Kirby.

Barry phoned to tell us he would be cancelling our purchase order. He was delighted to learn the helmet had already been shipped. It was now his. To show it around, however, would mean the end of his career.

The helmet sat in Barry's home for several months, then it fell off a table revealing its original red color. He called us and he was furious. He felt we had cheated him, then Bev explained the helmet was exactly what he had ordered — "just like the red one, only blue."

A year later when I was in Panama City on a sales trip, I contacted Barry and he invited me to his home for a wonderful dinner. He told me that the design of the Mark XII was not going well. I looked it over and, using a piece of butcher paper, I drew the best solution I could come up with. That new design was soon shipped to be constructed by Divex in New Orleans.

Another year passed and I was again visiting Panama City. Navy divers were evaluating the completed Mark XII system on the end of a concrete pier overlooking clear water with a bright sandy bottom. The troops were all wearing Mark XII T-shirts and carrying Mark XII gear bags. Everyone was hyped, agreeing with one another concerning the merits of the new diving system. Who could blame them? One negative word might land each man back on a destroyer escort, while duty in the tropics was very good and came with attractive, bikini-clad local ladies.

When a diver came up, he was asked a lot of questions including, "How's the visibility?"

"Oh shit, chief," he answered, "it's frigging great!"

"How was this?" and "How was that?" Every question was answered in the affirmative and with enthusiasm; there was not a word of negativity. I was reminded of the Hans Christian Anderson tale, "The King Was In His All Together." Everyone in the kingdom was admiring the king's wonderful outfit while, in fact, the king was nude.

The helmets and their associated equipment were then bid out. Morse of Boston won the contract and produced a slew of Mark XII systems, enough to outfit every ship and duty station in the navy. The size of the contract boggled our minds. We would never have a chance to handle such a large contract until many years had passed.

For perhaps twenty years, from 1976 until the mid-nineties, the Mark XII helmets and their associated gear lay in the back of diving lockers. Few saw duty, and those that did were buried even deeper the following day, in dark rooms filled with unneeded equipment. And, because the navy ends up with a new regime every twenty years, they were eventually declared obsolete and no more were ordered.

Our navy did turn out many excellent men, enlisted and officers. One such man was Captain George Bond, a submarine medical doctor who was the father of saturation diving.

Captain Bond continued with the theory that any tissue "saturates" with inert soluble breathing gas to a maximum limit at a given depth. Once saturated, the diver's decompression depth, the time needed for the gas in his tissues to come out of his tissues safely, is the same, regardless of the length of time he spends at that depth. Theoretically, a diver could live at depth if equipment were developed to support his existence and accomplish decompression. Pulling this off was not a small task.

Sometime around 1967, Washington got behind Bond and devised a plan to have divers live at great depths. The driving force behind this ambitious venture was the need to install equipment on the sea floor for offensive and defensive warfare, even though few understood the actual reasons for such a difficult project. Because of the high security required, the development of this type of underseas work could not be bid out to commercial operations such as Ocean Systems or Oceaneering. Years later, a book entitled *Blind Man's Bluff* was written on this subject, and it tells much of the story concerning divers in saturation doing "spook" work.

With the depth emphasis, the navy's Sea Lab program was conceived, and bids were let to proceed with the hardware. The Kirby Morgan Corporation was included, and we were hard put to make twelve Clamshell-style helmets, similar to those we made for John Harder and EDU.

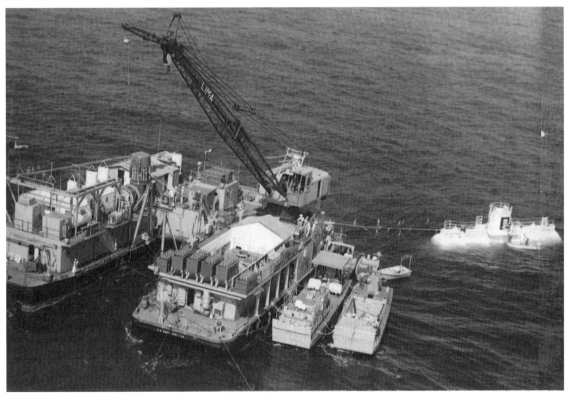

Paul Linaweaver

PLACING SEA LAB

In the meantime manned tests were to be conducted at Panama City. They would augment those planned for the extensive offshore concept test facility, Sea Lab, or Man Under the Sea Program. This operation was to be eventually located on the ocean floor off San Clemente Island at an ultimate depth of about 600 feet.

"Man in the Sea" windbreakers soon became the vogue at naval diving facilities, for the navy was extremely excited by the idea of putting men down in the ocean and having them live there.

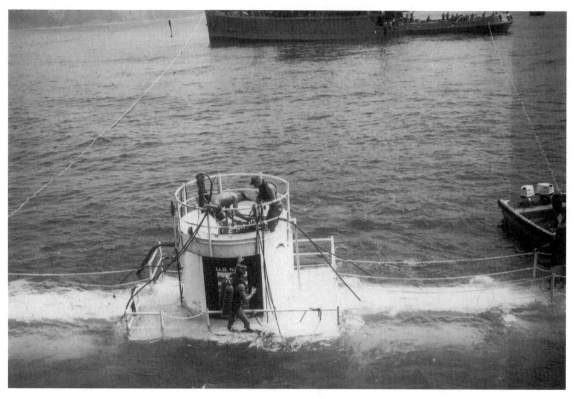

Paul Linaweaver

PLACING SEA LAB

This extensive plan, which would take place over a couple of years, included launching several diving operations, each deeper than the one before. It was an exciting time in naval diving history, and it was an exciting period for Bev and me as well.

As I mentioned earlier, the navy had their Mark VI recirculators (soon to be replaced by the Mark VIII and then the Mark IX), and all were designed for swimming. They were lung-powered; the diver's lung muscles would squeeze the gas from one bag into the other. En route, the gas was routed through a cleansing agent which removed the deadly carbon dioxide, a process similar to that of our heavy gear recirculator helmets. The lung-powered re-breathers used make-up oxygen. The gas was introduced in several different ways, with mechanical mass orifices or electronic metering, depending upon the style and age of the recirculators.

The diver breathed through a mouthpiece that was connected to two hoses, one for incoming gas and the other for outgoing. However, when his mouthpiece was in place the diver was totally handicapped and couldn't enunciate his words. This is where Bev and I came into the picture. Our new helmets would solve most of those problems, or so we hoped.

200

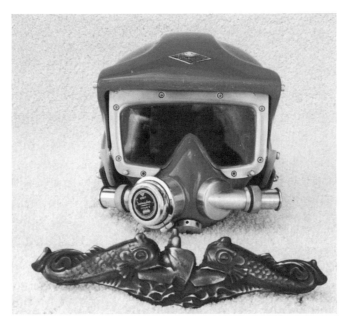

SEA LAB CLAMSHELL HELMET

Our new clamshell hats could not leak in any water or the carbon dioxide absorbent would fail. Beyond that, they had to retain the gas pressure from two bags, the same problem we had encountered in our two earlier naval contracts.

Our Sea Lab mission, to manufacture units that would work within these stringent limits, was a far more complex task than we had imagined at the time. Even more devastating, we would have to fund our research ourselves. Consequently, as we had no funds, we would be deploying very little research.

As I mentioned before, we had to design face seals that would retain the bag pressure; in addition, we were required to secure the units to the diver's head in a manner that defied any logical force to remove them. Then we discovered the inlet and outlet pipe diameters needed to be in excess of one inch to reduce breathing resistance, a challenge in itself. Also, the two rubber mushroom one-way valves had to be designed so that they would flow freely. Developing hardware for this alone would be costly.

Communications were essential, and the microphone location was critical. We also had to incorporate a view port that would provide the maximum field of vision plus an oral nasal mask to reduce CO_2 buildup while reducing internal volume. Lastly, we had to provide a means for purging unwanted water.

We were once again forced to build many more civilian masks in order to raise the necessary funds for our navy contract. Everyone assumed we were rolling in dough from our big Sea Lab contract; in fact, we were barely able to pay Skip Dunham, our one employee, a small salary, and we paid even less to ourselves. Our three-man team would be doing it all — civilian production and naval production — research, design, work, mold-making. There would be no vacations.

Our lack of funds became increasingly difficult to explain to our wives. (Women of little vision; they only wanted to pay the household bills. Women get so wound up in little details.) As it turned out, our money problems were the catalyst for our merger with Pacific Instruments. We needed bucks, and we needed them fast!

Our design eventually became known as the U.S. Navy Clamshell and, without dispute, it was the most beautiful diving helmet ever made. Unfortunately, its mechanical attributes did not measure up to its looks. The rear shell hinged on the top front of the retainer ring. The two rubber bungee cords that held it closed exerted a steady pressure against the back of the diver's skull which, as was the case with our SemiLite helmets, cut off the blood supply to the diver's head and generated a severe headache.

The front of each helmet was raised outward to clear the nose — referred to as the "beak" style — and the view port was notched to clear the beak. A nose-clearing device was not considered necessary as the diver was to don the rig inside a submerged habitat and remain at roughly the same depth for this entire dive.

All this was to be built at a cost of $1300 per helmet and, as I mentioned earlier, we had contracted to make twelve of them.

One reason it was so difficult to secure a decent contract at this time was because Captain Jacques Cousteau was dazzling the world with his underseas adventures. Wearing small yellow helmets with an antenna attached, his divers could be viewed swimming with fish in oceans around the world. The antenna allowed them to communicate with one another as easily as if they had been talking in a warm room. By the time the Sea Lab task was in motion, the adventures of Captain Cousteau were known to the world, and the men in Washington D.C. had also been watching him weekly on TV.

The truth was, Cousteau's yellow hats were fake and the antennas were bogus as well. His divers could not communicate with one another or with those topside. In order to provide an entertaining and believable television program, the underwater conversations were dubbed in at the studio. When we informed others of this they just blinked their eyes, for they believed what they saw. The powers in D.C. felt they would be funding us for research that had already been completed; they would be paying us to reinvent the wheel. All they wanted were helmets that worked as perfectly as those Cousteau and his men were wearing. Designing and building them was our problem. Did we want the work or not?

At six hundred feet, a diver's breathing gas is very dense. A diver in a habitat, doing hard work, soon becomes winded. The diameter of a man's windpipe is not large enough, and his lungs are not strong enough, to move a sufficient quantity of thick gas. Bev and I knew we could not increase the diameter of the windpipe, but we believed we could assist it by devising a method of pumping and then pulling the gas to and from his lungs at a slightly higher pressure. How much higher? And how to produce it? Answers to these questions remain mysteries to this day.

Our attempts at convincing others to research such a new horizon turned out to be a waste of time. Our meager funding could not begin to cover the cost. We were stuck with what we had, and so was the navy.

In order to achieve complete success, it was necessary to overcome three obstacles. First, the helmet design had to be advanced in style while remaining comfortable; second, a method had to be found to keep the diver warm; and third, a method had to be found to reduce diver breathing effort.

The challenge of keeping the diver warm was eventually solved by using hot water suits. Strange as this may seem, Sea Lab didn't use this complex but successful system, and their diver's froze out.

The breathing problem was never solved. All funding went toward the underwater living habitat, large vessels, barges, tugs, helicopters, jets, plane tickets, and administration overhead. Not a dime went toward research for diving helmets.

The "Man in the Sea" program was a worthy effort, however, for it proved that Dr. Bond's theories were correct. Unfortunately, his theories became political fodder. Astronaut Scott Carpenter was trained as the lead diver, and politicians arrived to reap the rewards by riding on the back of the high-profile project.

My departure from the Kirby Morgan Company in late 1968 carried me away from the final days of Sea Lab, but I continued to stay in touch with Bev. When the navy approached him for more Clamshell helmets, he replied with, "Sorry guys, they are pieces of crap. I won't build them anymore."

After Sea Lab came to an end, part of its saturation habitat ended up in front of the "Museum of Man in the Sea," a small museum in Panama City, Florida. Several of the Man in the Sea divers still live in Panama City, and they do their best to maintain it. They are a great bunch of men, perhaps the best part of the program. And Captain George Bond was probably the best of them all; a true pioneer and wonderful human being.

In 1969 Bev Morgan was again tasked to design and manufacture recirculator masks. Recalling the clamshell's problems, he decided to manufacture a new mask; one that was custom-fitted to the diver's face. However, the face seals interfered with the oral nasal masks that were standard on the line of Band Masks Bev had sold to U.S. Divers. In order to clear the new face seal, he decided to reshape the oral nasal mask so that it fit high on the diver's chin instead of under it. His hard work paid off, for his recirculator masks withstood the pressure. Communications were good, and the masks were quite comfortable. The money continued to flow, allowing my former partner to concentrate on the Band Mask's many problems.

In 1970 U.S. Divers had not only purchased the Band Mask line from Bev but, in order to reduce production costs, had also retooled it. As a result, quality was affected and fewer masks were purchased each month. Because Bev was receiving royalty for each unit sold, he grew anxious. After proper lobbying, however, U.S. Divers was successful in getting the navy to adopt the Band Mask as its standard diving equipment for shallow water underseas tasks including hull repair.

The naval lab in Panama City designed a new side valve assembly for the units with a much better flow rate. They had the mask's plastic parts cast in black, instead of orange, and named the units "USN MK I MOD 0 Diver's Mask."

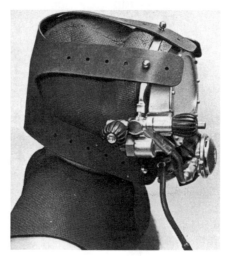

U.S. NAVY MARK I

Over the years our naval troops in Panama City came to believe their engineers at the lab had designed the entire mask. This fantasy grew until it included the story that Bev and I were thieves; two unscrupulous individuals who had stolen the designs from the navy and then marketed them. Actually, the improved side valve was the only part of the Band Mask that had been designed by the navy and, at that time, U.S. Divers, a French firm, owned the design, not Kirby or Morgan.

During a visit to Florida in 1976, I was sitting at a conference table when a chief accused me of stealing ideas, including the Mark I mask, from the U.S. Navy. I was then ushered out the front gate, assisted by an armed guard. The red-faced chief who had leveled the accusation was quite sincere in his beliefs, and I was never invited back.

Once the navy contracted with U.S. Divers for the Mark I, more changes were made by the military. This was a little like taking pills; if one is good, two must be better.

They did not want to use our inexpensive paper speakers; they were considered to be "Mickey Mouse" by the naval lab engineers. Still, these speakers worked very well and, as I said, they were cheap. The navy got together with U.S. Divers and ordered "lollipop" speakers, encapsulated in urethane. These were far more expensive but, according to the U.S. Divers sales pitch, they were waterproof and would last forever. However, they failed completely.

Once a thing was navy-approved, no force on earth could change the design. Naval diving stations were not allowed to purchase speakers that actually worked, and this single problem — a lack of communications with topside — rendered the Mark I useless.

Compounding their error, U.S. Divers decided that if the urethane lollipop speakers were good enough for the navy, they were just the thing for their civilian masks as well. As a result, the Band Mask line began to falter and Bev's royalties fell even further.

The upturned oral nasal masks that Bev had designed for the recirculator masks soon made their way to U.S. Divers as well. Not understanding that they were shaped to clear a water-filled face seal, U.S. Divers adopted the new oral nasal shape for the civilian Band Masks and the Navy's Mark I. This was a disaster because the divers experienced extreme discomfort. Just like the worthless speakers, they were navy approved. One more nail was driven into the coffin of the Mark I design.

Over the years, more and more Mark I masks did shelf-side duty in lockers at the navy's diving stations. What good is a mask that provides no better communications than scuba? Without reliable communications with topside, the navy was no better off than it had been with the Jack Browne masks, twenty years earlier. The naval scuba rigs soon won out, and the Mark I was judged obsolete.

Meanwhile, commercial diving firms had reinstalled the paper speakers in their band masks, and with good results. Other firms supplied proper oral nasal masks to replace the small ones. The Band Mask soon became a successful mainstay, as did the DSI Heliox 18, a similar design that we at DSI were making.

Underwater construction mandates good communications topside. Without this, a task takes longer and is much more dangerous. For this very reason, commercial diving firms such as Oceaneering and the Association of Diving Contractors have banned scuba.

As time went by, more and more commercial diving firms were invited to bid on jobs that had formerly been accomplished by navy diving teams. Eventually, the naval diving operations lost a large portion of underseas work. Because of their reluctance to look around and possibly change their way of doing things, our navy shot itself in the foot. Little has changed since I was a sailor.

In the early days of commercial saturation diving, everyone considered the possibility of recirculating the gas from the diver to the surface for scrubbing before sending it back to the bell. This concept is known as the "push-pull system." The plan was simple enough; the hardware with which to accomplish it was complex. That is, until Allen Crasburg succeeded where others had tried and failed.

Taylor Diving of New Orleans had engaged in an effort based on the Swindell helmet, a rather buoyant hat designed with straps and cables to secure it to the diver. It could be mated to a breastplate and a standard dress as well, but it was usually used as swim gear with a neck dam, much like the navy's Mark XII.

Taylor designers built a can on the helmet's rear. It incorporated a large diaphragm and a spool valve which was sealed with two O-rings. Should the helmet experience a slight internal over-pressure, the diaphragm would bulge outward, sliding the spool valve outward and opening a port to topside. An internal under-pressure would slide the valve closed. All this seemed very simple on paper.

In the field, sliding O-rings can be fickle. Sometimes they slide and sometimes they don't. During a test dive the valve slid open but did not close, and the diver experienced a severe under-pressure and was squeezed into his helmet. Taylor scrapped the project, but some of their many employees were old navy divers. Word quickly spread to the Panama City lab and the lab called Taylor. They wanted to buy a push-pull system for testing, and Taylor complied.

The navy now possessed a topside recirculating system which did not work. In fact it could be deadly. In order to experiment with the system, a complete facility was set up across the road from the Experimental Diving Unit. Although test after test confirmed the inherent problem, the navy's engineers knew a good thing when they saw it. As I said earlier, Panama City duty was as good as it gets. The program lasted six years at a staggering cost before it was finally abandoned.

After rejoining Bev and forming DSI in 1974, we eventually ended up with the SuperLite 17, an all-time winner. In 1976 I was invited to the Mare Island sub base in Vallejo to demonstrate it. I was greeted by Lieutenant Peter Faucet who informed me he had heard great things about our little swim hats. He had been informed they kept a diver's head dry, afforded great communications, and employed the best breathing regulator in the industry. In this case, Peter was well-informed.

I always began my demonstrations by doing something very stupid. This demonstration began with my Captain Jet, "arms to the side," dive into the water (I preferred performing this stunt off a diving board rather than a bar stool); a maneuver which always appeared to impress the troops. (Of course, any other diver executing this stunt on the job would have been fired, and I would have been the first to let him go.)

Unfortunately, the lower board at the large naval pool had been removed so, in order to live up to the reputation that had preceded me, I was duty-bound to make my big splash from the upper board, twelve feet over the water. I came close to breaking my neck in the process, but I did make the sale!

Peter Faucet bought one hat and then did his best to introduce the design into the ranks of his divers and those at other naval diving duty stations as well. When his efforts succeeded in only raising eyebrows, he discovered that being a lieutenant in the navy is no big deal. He was ordered to forget the SuperLite 17 and return to the use of regulation navy gear; that is unless he wanted to end up manning that lighthouse in Greenland, a duty that Commander Barry Ridgewell narrowly escaped.

Ten years would pass before Chief Powell, in San Diego, put his job on the line and succeeded in having the navy adopt the SuperLite 17, one of the best moves Uncle Sam ever made. And Powell was probably successful only because he knew people in the right places, including an admiral who pulled the correct strings.

One day in 1978 we received a phone call from a group of army divers in Newport News, Virginia. They wanted a demonstration of the SuperLite 17, so off I went. Their operation was run by a master sergeant who had a small diving company on the side. My demonstration was well-received, and I was asked to leave the hat for further testing and evaluation. When I called my home office, I was advised the helmet was to return home with me. Once I was back in California, I rounded up all the blemished SuperLite 17 parts I could find, and I built a hat minus a serial number; in fact, the hat itself was non-existent. Then I sent it to the master sergeant as a gift with the understanding that my act of kindness was to be kept between the two of us. Later, for reasons then unknown to Skip or Bev, the army ordered many SuperLite 17. I am writing this today to enlighten Bev as to the army's acceptance of our DSI helmets.

Several years later, in the east, an airliner slid off the end of a runway in the winter, and many passengers ended up in the freezing river. The navy was tasked to salvage the wreck and recover the bodies. Once in the water, the inlet valves of their Mark XII rigs froze shut. The army's diving team from Newport News showed up with their SuperLites and accomplished the task. The navy responded by ordering the army to quit using the DSI hats until they had been approved by the navy. The master sergeant told the navy to go to hell, and the army continued to use the 17. Now there was a good man. I liked him from the start.

By 1976, Diving Systems had redesigned the Band Mask using hand-laid fiberglass instead of injection-molded plastic. The new design was called the Heliox 18, and it was a very good unit. We did our darndest to get the navy to adopt them in place of the obsolete, Mark I which had been supplied by U.S. Divers. As I said earlier, U.S. Divers was French-owned, and it was a legal no no for our government to be purchasing equipment from a foreign country if the same or equivalent product could be built in the USA.

Lobbyists do have their ways. "Hey, Captain Mickelson, where the hell are you today? And did you ever recover from that last dose of clap, asshole?."

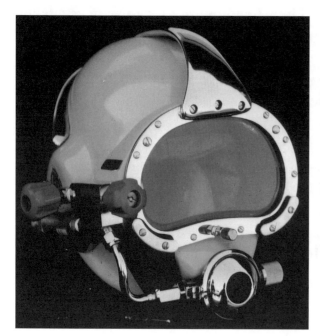 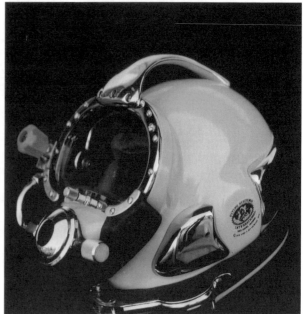

SUPERLITE 17

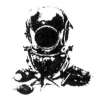

DIVING SYSTEMS INTERNATIONAL

Jack Conroy went broke in 1971, and my job as an aircraft mechanic disappeared. I worked for a few other aviation firms but they eventually suffered the same fate. I then returned to pile driving but, because of my fair skin, the sun was once again my enemy. It became obvious I would have to resume my talents in the diving helmet business or we would starve. I remembered how I had helped to found the Kirby Morgan Corporation in 1965, and wondered if there was a way Bev and I could do it again.

One night I awakened from a dream and recalled my cousin, Lester Dresser, who owned what was probably the world's poorest dairy just north of Sacramento. When I was a youngster, my mother and I spent several summers there. Milking the cows and attending to the various chores was hard, but the tiring work was punctuated with a cool swim every day in the Sacramento River.

The summer I was twelve, girls began to draw my attention. I pretended not to notice them until one, she was probably around fifteen, swam by in a white transparent shirt. The following summer I pleaded to return to the dairy and my mother, unaware of my motives, gave in. I resumed my duties as a dairyman, but the girl in the transparent shirt was never seen again.

Lester was very lean, strong as a bull but thin enough to almost be blown away. One day he crept up behind me and, placing his cupped hands under my jaw, he lifted me off the ground by my head. I screamed and kicked until his arms gave in to my thirteen years of accumulated weight. When I awakened, still groggy, from my dream years later, I recalled this event. I didn't remember my cousin's treatment as particularly painful, and I wondered...was there a way to design a diving helmet that could be secured to the head in the same manner? Was it possible for a helmet to be cupped under the jaws and at the back of the head instead of using a chin strap? Because dreams have a habit of disappearing by morning, I leaped out of bed and scribbled down my thoughts. (Claudia muttered a few words about my being crazy before rolling over.)

The next morning the notes I had jotted down still made sense, and the summer of 1974 was the summer I invented the "yoke," a new method of helmet retention. I built a crude prototype and attached it to a helmet I constructed from a design Bev had discarded earlier. This was the same little red hat we would later sell to Barry Ridgewell.

Two days later I knocked on the door of Bev's Santa Barbara shop. He had moved from the airport to a rusting corrugated iron building behind the Diver's Den, and he invited me in. I immediately spotted several models of swim helmets sitting on top of a high shelf that ran the length of the wall — designs that Bev had developed since we parted in 1968 but had never put into production. I could guess why; while the helmets were handsome, none possessed the final necessary ingredient — a decent method of retention.

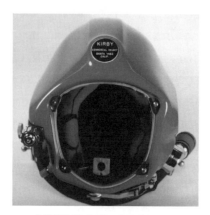

LITTLE RED HELMET

When Bev tried on my little air hat, he was immediately inspired. "Bob," he said, "can I have five percent of the yoke design?"

"No Bev," I told him. "You can have fifty."

We became equal partners once again, but we were as broke as ever. We felt as if we might be onto something, but we had no idea that we would be developing our own new company — Diving Systems International.

Bev needed money as badly as me; customers were no longer ordering deep diving face seals, and his only other source of income were the Band Mask royalties from U.S. Divers, and they had almost ceased.

As we held the little swim hat in our arms, we pondered our next move. After test-diving it in the Diver's Den pool, Bev emerged elated. He had a plan. We would sell our prototype to the navy.

Bev then reluctantly informed me that he had promised a military acquaintance from the spook group a one-half interest in his manufacturing business if he ever got back into production. His friend, a naval deep operations officer, was a tall thin, obviously educated and well-mannered gentleman; in short — a very polished individual. Claiming to be a mover and a shaker, he had presented Bev with a well-documented resume. He was to muster out in the immediate future, and he appeared to be just the man to head a manufacturing plant upon his return to civilian life.

One of Bev's long handles is that his word is as good as a contract. Since he had promised this man a position in his future manufacturing endeavors, that is how it would have to be. I had a choice of either going along or of scrapping the project, and I reluctantly agreed to join them. Still, there was something about the gentleman that bothered me; I just couldn't put my finger on it.

As soon as Barry Ridgewell had our free flow hat, now painted blue, and we had the navy's $5000, the three of us began working on a second model, a model outfitted with a very sophisticated servo demand regulator.

As had been the case before, designing this regulator turned out to be much more difficult than we had anticipated. We also had to hand-feed our new partner helmet theories and designs which further complicated matters. We were actually dragging him along, kicking and arguing all the way. Then he suddenly decided he had conceived the new design himself, and he proceeded to tell the world. It was as if Bev and I didn't exist. He was quickly becoming a thorn in my side.

He had done a handsome job gaining Bev's confidence, however, and he enjoyed Bev's respect. I'm sure this was because Bev knew me only too well, while our partner was a new boy on the block. Lacking a formal education and sporting old Levis, I was certainly no competition for this educated, retired military officer who still dressed the part.

Dick Quittner and his machining talents did not come cheap. We needed money to complete the servo regulator, and our partner came to our rescue. "I have $7000 in the bank," he told us, "and all I'm receiving is interest. Say the word and it's yours. Pay me back when you can."

The day of reckoning arrived. I had run up a handsome fee with Mr. Quittner, and our machinist was as badly in need of cash as Bev and I. When we told our partner we needed a couple thousand, he assured us he would have the money the following day. There was, however, a new consideration. In addition to his original share in the manufacturing firm, he now wanted a third of our new yoke patent. If we didn't want to take him up on this, he was withdrawing his funding offer. Expressing no shame or emotion, it was simply business as usual.

Bev phoned me that evening. "Is it my imagination, or is he as ruthless as he appears to be?" After assuring Bev that our partner lacked business ethics, I suggested he be eliminated from our company as quickly as possible. Bev asked me to show up early the following morning. I didn't know what he was up to, but I imagined it would be something spectacular for I had seen him in action before.

Bev and I were enjoying our coffee as the minute hand ticked away. Before long, we heard a key slide into the lock. The door opened and there he stood, well-dressed as usual, holding his leather briefcase in one hand, his keys in the other, and smiling as if he had already succeeded with his corporate takeover. He did not know Bev Morgan.

Bev asked him to pull up a chair. He did not offer him a cup of coffee, for the man would not be present long enough to drink it. "Open your briefcase," Bev told him. He placed his briefcase on the floor and opened it. "Now," Bev continued, "turn it upside down and dump the contents on the floor." After he had complied, Bev looked him in the eyes and said, "Remove any items that belong to you."

The polished former officer fumbled nervously through the stack of assorted pens, pocket calculators, and papers as he gathered his own things. "Now, please close your briefcase and leave. Don't ever come back. We never want to see you again."

After our former partner had left the office, Bev sat in silence, contemplating our need for $2000. I handed him a check, for Claudia had agreed to loan us most of the savings she and I had accumulated. Like me, Claudia had not trusted our ex-partner from the moment she met him. Claudia was an excellent judge of character.

It soon became clear to Bev and I that our new helmet, outfitted with the wonderful servo regulator, was not going to work. The steady flow helmet we had sold to the navy earlier was a much better design but, before it could be accepted by the industry, it needed a regulator.

We decided to scrap the servo demand hat and replace it with something more practical that would be readily received. Bev came up with a marketing plan that, looking back, was not a necessarily good idea. (To put this in perspective, my own list of mistakes is much longer than Bev's.)

We would manufacture the Kirby Morgan 16, a dry helmet shell that could mate to an existing Band Mask, thus converting the mask into a dry helmet. The strategy was great, but the helmet's design was complex.

The helmet had a waterproof bladder that clamped under the band of the Band Mask and was secured to the hard fiberglass shell with a similar clamp. A heavy brass casting, for both weight and helmet retention, acted as the yoke and was clamped onto the bottom of the shell with metal clips. It soon became known in the industry as "the design from hell."

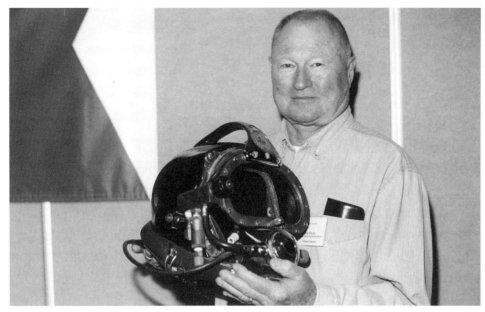

KIRBY MORGAN 16

After viewing the prototype, Dennis Jady, Dan Wilson's top man at Sub Sea International, ordered several. Before we could even begin to complete them, we ran out of money again. This time Bev offered to mortgage his home and asked me to do the same. Because I owed more on our new home than it was worth, I had to refuse. Bev now owned well over half of our new corporation while I retained fifteen percent; a huge drop from half, but he who finances, controls. This is a fact of life.

We rehired Skip Dunham, who had left Bev in 1971, and Tom Protheroe who was a friend of mine from my aircraft days. Tom would be our new mold maker and also do the lay-up work. I did most of the mechanical assembly. Bev took care of all the business matters.

This complex helmet was not well received at Sub Sea International because it was easy to drop the brass yoke from a saturation bell during the dressing in procedure. Pressure was on for us to come up with something better, and very soon.

The task of designing a new helmet is very demanding. It requires time and money, and it took us over a year, and several prolonged attempts, to develop the SuperLite 17. In the meantime we needed another financial bandage. We decided to manufacture a Band Mask look-alike using fiberglass, as in our original, instead of the injection-molded ABS plastic used by U.S. Divers, and we named it the Heliox 18 Mask. It was a fine product. We had made a very good move.

Orders began to arrive, and it soon became apparent that we needed a larger facility. Bev located a building in Santa Barbara on Laguna Street with a small office and a large open warehouse that had been occupied by a roofing company. We managed to purchase it with a minimal down payment and small regular payments, something that could never take place today. As I've mentioned before, Bev was no fool when it came to business and real estate.

The shop building, perhaps four thousand square feet, was basically useless because there was no electricity, so Tom Protheroe had to work outside and run extension cords from outlets within the office. We not only needed to maintain our present production but, anticipating production increases, we obviously needed to improve our facility.

I was selected to wire the entire shop and, in light of Santa Barbara's stringent building codes and generally negative attitude concerning manufacturers, this would be a formidable task. Both Tom and I had taken up soaring as a hobby, and I approached one of the soaring club members, Jim Day, owner of Day Electric in Lompoc and a bona fide electrical contractor, for help.

"It's simple," he told me. "All we have to do is draw up an electrical load schedule. This is an electrical map, and it is a requirement if you want a permit. I'll be glad to help. How you get it through the planning department is your problem."

Bill Painter, another club member, was a builder and he knew the local ropes. When I explained our need to install electricity and make several other structural changes, he told me to forget it. "The building is within the coastal zone. There's a moratorium on building, and you'll never be issued a permit. My advice is to sell the place."

I was sick over this news, but I considered his advice. The next day I put on tattered Levis and a denim shirt smeared with fiberglass resin; then I ran a rope through the belt loops. Now I looked and smelled like a surfboard maker.

Pushing through the weathered metal door of the building inspector's office, I got in line. A small balding man stood behind the counter and sitting on this counter was his name engraved on a rectangular wooden nameplate.

"Hi," I said, affecting a thick southern drawl, "I'm Bob Kirby." Reluctantly, he took my out-held hand and shook it. "We have rented an old building on Laguna Street," I told him, "and it don't got no electricity so we have extension cords kinda running to it. The problem is cars run over the cords and cut them, causing fires and things like that. What can we do to fix it?"

The county worker turned from me in disgust. (And did I detect him swearing under his breath?) Then, in phrases slow and precise enough to be understood by a patient with advanced Alzheimer's, he told me I would have to make out a load schedule. "A licensed Santa Barbara electrical contractor MUST do this. Do you understand?"

I nodded.

"Then you will have to return and we will evaluate it. IF we approve it, an electrical contractor must install the wiring. Do you understand?"

Thanking him with all my heart and pumping his hand in appreciation (probably against his wishes) I returned to our office where I composed a letter to his supervisor stating that the most helpful individual in all Santa Barbara County had waited on me. I wrote that he was a credit to the building department and to its supervisor. I ended with "Thank God for people like yourself who will take the time to help someone like me." I signed my letter, "Bob Kirby, surfboard maker."

The following day Jim Day and I drew up the load schedule on a large sheet of butcher paper. Using a wide pencil, we made many mistakes which we erased and corrected. I crumpled the paper up, stood on it, poured coffee on it and then, as a final touch, I smeared a bit of fiberglass resin on it. I was off to the building inspector's office to revisit the little bald man behind the counter.

He saw me coming and actually ran to meet me. Holding out his hand in a gesture of friendship, he welcomed me. "It's good to see you again. Let me see your load schedule. Wow. It's a little rough. Oh well, I'll go back and run a calculation on the loads."

I could hear his fingers running over the calculator like a mouse in a can of walnuts; then he emerged with a broad smile. "Well, Bob," he said, "the loads are great. Hold on while I make out a permit. We'll need a check for $200."

The Heliox 18 was doing well. We equipped it with regulators made by U.S. Divers for their Band Mask line; regulators we had purchased from U.S. Divers dealers across the country. By 1976, the French firm was considering us to be serious competition, so U.S. Divers would not sell regulators to us directly. Eventually, when the cat was completely out of the bag, U.S. Divers stopped production of all regulators except those needed by their own company. I was completing the design of our SuperLite prototype when Skip Dunham, our new president, informed me we could no longer purchase demand regulators, and we were forced to manufacture them ourselves — and within six weeks.

After un-soldering a U.S. Divers regulator, we took the parts to Dick Quittner at Experimental Machine and asked him to make them. Then a strange thing happened. Our old friend declined the work unless we extended him an open agreement to do all our machine work from then on.

I ended up visiting machine shops, door to door. Rich Watkins, owner of Aero Machine Goleta, took on the entire line at a much better price. A local metal stamping house, PK Engineering, produced our new levers that were outfitted with rollers. Ours was an improvement over the U.S. Divers design— and a big one. I located a deep-draw stamping plant that could make the cans, covers, and snap rings.

The stamping plant was in the bowels of Culver City and, because I was visiting it during the Watts riots, I bought myself a small automatic handgun before my meeting with Mr. Cooper, the owner. The windows of the once-proud shop were covered with sheets of plywood, and I wasn't sure I had the right address until a little old man, accompanied by a large black dog, answered the door and introduced himself.

Mr. Cooper was a true gentleman and one hell of a machinist. His critter was an honest-to-goodness junkyard dog that had been laying against oily machinery since birth. Unfortunately, the dog was friendly and when he cuddled up to me he made a mess of my for-once clean trousers.

During the assembly of the regulators, a young man by the name of Pete Ryan rode in from the east coast on a motorcycle. He was looking for a job and took on the task of soldering and quality checking the regulators. Pete is still running Diving Systems research and development division today.

I continued with the design of the SuperLite 17, and I did a long list of production tasks including tooling for the drilling of the many holes in the fiberglass frames and tooling for the bending of many metal parts and several welding fixtures. Though those of us in research and development were up to our ears in projects, these were especially good times.

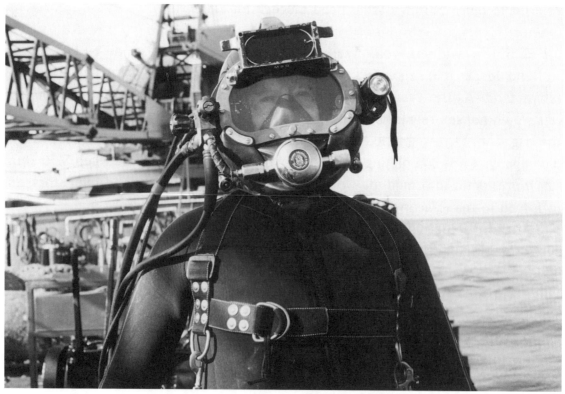

Mike San Gabriel
GENE AISWORTH, SUPERLITE 17, GAVIOTA, 2000

The SuperLite turned out to be winner, and we hired a second fiberglass laminator who was as good as they come. Unfortunately, he had a history of drugs and, though he perished

216

after overdosing sometime later, Jimmy was with us for several years.

Bev's demeanor had changed since the days when we were equal partners in our Kirby Morgan Corporation. In retrospect, I understand why. During the interim years I had formed Conroy Aircraft Corporation in Goleta, a firm with over 100 employees. I had been running that firm in ways that were totally different from those when Bev was in charge. Meanwhile, Bev had continued as his own boss, changing his ways of doing business as the need arose.

We were both carrying baggage when we rejoined forces; my aircraft corporation had gone under after a major crash in Alaska, while problems with U.S. Divers and Uncle Sam left Bev with severe wounds. Back together again, each of us assumed the other was on his wavelength. But, of course, we were not. Too much water had passed under our bridges for us to be as compatible as we had been during the Kirby Morgan days. And before my involvement with Diving Systems International was over, we would have irreparable differences. Our eventual separation was unavoidable. For the time being, however, we were managing to get along and we were making money.

Once a year, Diving Systems attended the Association of Diving Contractors symposium in either New Orleans or Houston. Skip, Bev and I would attend, setting up our booth and manning it. Although it appeared as if we were on a vacation, this was extremely hard and demanding work. As we manned our booth each day, even though we were bone tired, we would try to stay in good spirits. We would take clients out to dinner in the evening, get rather drunk and, nursing splitting headaches, we would have to do it over again the next day.

One year while attending a symposium in New Orleans we stayed at the prestigious Hyatt Regency Hotel. As usual, we spent a couple of days setting up our booth; then, when it was operational, the three of us went to dinner and Bev came up with a ploy to fool our accountant, just for the fun of it. Instead of billing each room for expenses, the three of us would use my room number for the tab. The end result would be the same, for Diving Systems International would pay for everything. Our joke would simplify accounting and should have pleased our accounting department. It did not.

Our head accountant went over all the invoices, then pulled me into her office and demanded an explanation. "You are one expensive date," she told me. "Your tab is seven times Bev's and Skip's. I guess you had a good time in New Orleans. Perhaps you'll take me along next time, or I'll tell." When I attempted to explain the situation, she refused to listen.

Shortly after leaving Diving Systems International, I dropped in for a visit and noticed another accountant now occupied the previous accountants desk. When I asked about her, Skip told me to keep it down. "She is a difficult subject around here." I badgered Skip until he told me the particulars.

Bev was going over the books one day when he noticed that the accountant had purchased numerous airline tickets for trips she and her husband had enjoyed. When he confronted her, she told him that Bob Kirby had enjoyed a very expensive outing in New Orleans. She was simply taking her share.

Another Association of Divers Contractors symposium in Houston had a perhaps more humorous outcome. Skip and I had been working our booth, demonstrating the SuperLite 17 to any diver who wished to view it. Occasionally, there was standing room only. Ben Miller, a helmet manufacturer from Texas, came into our booth. "Bob," he said, "I have to go to the head in a bad way. Will you man my booth in my absence?"

"No problem," I told him. "I'm on my way."

Soon the same gaggle of divers made their way to Benny Miller's booth where I was now seated. "Didn't we just see you in DSI's booth?" one asked.

"Oh yes, you did," I exclaimed.

"Why are you here?" was the next question.

"Because these helmets are very good." I dropped it at that. They departed, scratching both their heads and their rear ends.

Bev and I began butting heads over mechanical designs. He would give me an assignment and I would dive into its problems with both feet, moving forward as fast as possible. In order to accomplish the design criteria, considerable changes were sometimes necessary, and Bev's original theme would have been abandoned. Every couple of weeks he would come in to inspect my progress and, often as not, the direction I was taking strayed from his original concept. I felt these changes were necessary but Bev, who disagreed, would take the task home for evaluation.

He seldom brought them back and, at one point, fifteen projects which I had outlined disappeared. Eventually, I was no longer doing research.

To produce a saleable product there are several requirements; an R and D arm, manufacturing tooling and, eventually, sales and management. By now our tooling was in poor repair, and Bev hated the day-by-day manufacturing process with its ongoing problems. He never stood in my way of making new tools; in fact he never scrutinized them after they were finished. Consequently, I immersed myself in the problems manufacturing had to offer.

And I amazed myself. After three months of redoing the mechanical tooling, I was able to reduce assembly time by half. Unfortunately, I was then out of work, so I repeated the scenario and reduced the assembly time by an additional ten percent. But after working in the shop and dealing with production problems exclusively, I grew short-tempered and moody. Bev was picking up on my bursts of anger, but he kept it to himself.

I began to experience periods of depression and, after a time, I started to feel as if electrical shocks were being transmitted through my head. These shocks might take place several times a day and, if I was driving, I could only hold on and pray, frozen to the wheel, until the seizure passed. I was in such stress one night that I thought I was dying and was admitted to emergency. I was having what appeared to be a nervous breakdown.

My doctor, Dr. Van Valin, prescribed a tranquilizer that I was to take daily. Over the months, the dosage was gradually reduced. Though I was eventually pronounced out of the woods, I was no longer able to handle any pressure, with or without tranquilizers. I would simply fall apart. In 1980, two years after my departure from Diving Systems International, my eyesight began to fail, and a large brain tumor was discovered in my pituitary gland. The tumor had been there for some time. I had not been able to handle pressure because my body had not been producing adrenaline. The tumor, pressing on my optic nerves, had also reduced my vision. Once the tumor was removed, my sight returned.

We received a call from an Englishman who had invented a gas return valve that the dive industry needed. When it arrived, I hooked it up to a mask, and Skip and I test dove it in my swimming pool. The design was amazing. There was absolutely no bubble noise and no exhaust back-pressure. We received word the inventor was on his way and would arrive in Santa Barbara the following Saturday.

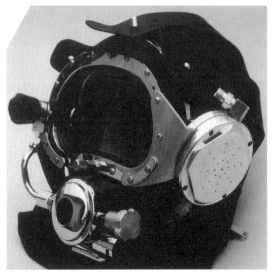

GAS RETURN VALVE ON OUR MASK

For some time, Bev had been bragging about his celebrity friend, David Crosby. "You should see Crosby's new Mercedes. It's a 450 SEL, perhaps the finest car made."

Saturday, the day the Englishman would be arriving, I borrowed Dr. Van Valin's limousine, a long, black, 1962 Mercedes 600 that had been built for the Queen of England. I knew the doctor had paid over $100,000 for it — probably twice the amount Crosby had paid for his machine.

There has never been a more beautiful automobile. Gazing onto its hand-rubbed lacquered finish was like looking into a pool of oil. The interior carpet was cobalt blue, and the limo had rich leather seating, inlaid hardwood paneling, a television set, and a bar.

I timed my entrance to coincide with the English gentleman's arrival and Bev was talking to him as I drove by. Behind the wheel of my long, sleek beast, I nudged up to the two of them. Bev was as mad as I had expected him to be, but he played it cool. The only thing our guest could say was, "What a car. What a car." I never heard another word about Crosby's Mercedes.

In the spring of 1980, soon after the limousine incident, I was fired. Not because of my practical joke, but because of the months Bev had endured my hostile behavior. He had had enough of me, and I didn't blame him.

He provided me with a very liberal termination agreement; much better than I expected. I agreed to a clause specifying five years of non-competition, and I was to be paid off for my share in our corporate property and would be receiving monthly payments for ten years. I was to also receive a royalty check for each helmet's retail sales price and for the balance of the patent's life. I would be receiving a very handsome amount some months, so I had little to complain about. Still, I had been fired from a firm I had helped to found, and this was difficult to accept. The name Kirby Morgan was synonymous with all the things I loved. On the other hand, I expect no other solution was possible. We had each extended ourselves to the limit.

I accepted a job offer from Whitey Stefens at Ocean Systems, and we built a 150-foot diving and work-over ship in Long Beach. I was the welding foreman and had the privilege of training my oldest son, Jeff, as a shipfitter. Those five months of hard physical labor improved my mood tremendously. We were proud of our accomplishments, and Whitey became one of my best friends.

After working at Ocean Systems, I was hired to teach commercial diving and related subjects at Santa Barbara City College where, after two years, my poor education and an inability to spell led to my termination.

I followed my teaching career with a job as an engineer (minus a degree) for Western Space and Marine of Santa Barbara.

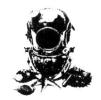

WESTERN SPACE AND MARINE

One day in 1983 Greg Bryant stepped into my office at Santa Barbara City College. After offering to buy me lunch he added, "I'll take you to meet Scott Millard who owns Western Space and Marine. Scott takes on all sorts of projects. His last project was to bore a hole in an iceberg in order to secure a towing eye into the mass, then tow it free of the shipping lanes."

Scott Millard's shop was the former Helms Bakery on Santa Barbara Street, one short block from the ocean. The brick and wood building had seen better days, and its corrugated tin roof leaked. The interior was a patchwork of plywood, two by fours and other small scraps of wood. In an effort to cover the many cracks and poor workmanship, the walls had been repainted many times. On a more positive note, the rent was low.

When we entered, the shop's imposing owner was on the telephone. This, I was to discover, was his favorite pastime. His full white beard danced up and down in time with his jaw, and his large stomach prevented him from sitting close to his desk which was piled high with paper and miscellaneous other items.

When Scott replaced the phone and turned to face us, his broken-down swivel chair complained loudly. He was smiling, or so it seemed, and his beard was even fuller than it had appeared when viewed from behind. When he stood up and shook my hand, I felt as if I might be a long-lost brother. At that instant a friendship was formed that continues to this day. I certainly had no idea that this introduction would lead to some of the most exciting − and occasionally bizarre − experiences in my life.

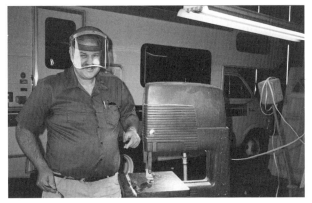

SCOTT MILLARD

My impending dismissal from City College was welcome news to Scott. He had recently sold two manipulator arms to the navy to be used on the *Turtle*, a small manned submersible stationed in San Diego to be refitted. General Electric had originally designed the arms; designing and selling are two different matters, however, and GE had failed in the latter. After many years and numerous sales attempts, GE had sold the entire project to Scott. These two arms were to be Scott's first.

Delivery lead time was nine months and, in the meantime, the navy needed a mockup to assure adequate clearance for a vast array of added outside hardware. This mockup constructed of wood, fiberglass, and metal was to be full-sized; almost six feet long. It would be built with fake hydraulic cylinders that appeared to drive rack and pinion gears on sealed shafts with a mocked-up metal gripper on the arm's end. The mockup was to be a carbon copy of the real McCoy.

Scott was having trouble finding a good model maker and asked if I would accept employment. I agreed and would begin to work for him the day after I left City College. Because the work area in Scott's shop was open to both his engineering department and his machine shop, sawdust and fiberglass grindings would find their way into the smallest places, so I offered to build the mockup in my own shop. Though my wooden barn was full of spiders and holes, it was well-suited for such a grubby task. Scott gave me carte blanche and one very challenging month in which to complete the project.

He stopped in my shop once a week and, at first, most of the many required pieces were in a rough state, scattered all over the place. It didn't appear as if I was making progress but, one month to the day, I arrived at his facility with the completed mockup. Scott had a difficult time believing his eyes, for the mockup looked like the real thing — right down to the smallest bolts, nuts, and hydraulic hoses. When he delivered it to the navy, they thought it was the real arm.

Our mockup served its intended purpose. After the *Turtle* refit the model was transferred to a navy display case where it still resides some twenty years later. This initial success sealed my future with my new friend.

During the construction of the two *Turtle* arms, Scott hired my youngest son, Troy, as a fledgling machinist. Then Scott's senior machinist, a man who continually argued with his boss and was tired of the project, quit. Troy was left in charge. All of us were somewhat concerned until God came to our aid in the guise of Jerry Phillips. Jerry had retired as head machinist at General Motors Aerospace in Goleta, but he had grown bored with retirement and needed a part-time job.

I had fun observing this team; the old man and the kid. Jerry knew what he was doing, and Troy appreciated Jerry sharing his background and offering his extensive knowledge. Sometimes it was difficult to determine who was in charge, but it really didn't matter because our machine parts were accurately made and they arrived on time.

222

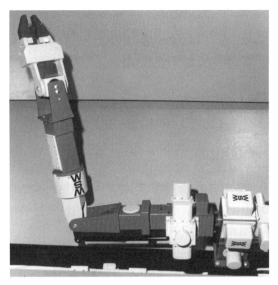

MOCKUP ARM FOR THE TURTLE

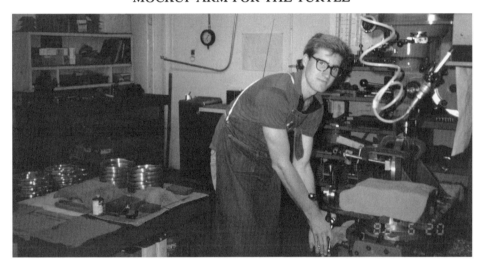

TROY MACHINING THE NECK RINGS

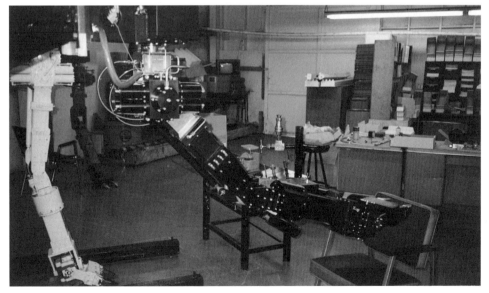

REAR ARM FOR THE TURTLE, 1987

223

Before we had completed the two arms Scott received a call from the navy lab in Panama City, Florida. Jim Middleton had heard I was now working at Western Space and Marine, and the navy wanted a SuperLite 17 modified to accept a re-breather for deep diving. We agreed on a price not to exceed $10,000.

Then an unfortunate situation took place, for Jim Middleton had his number-one man call Diving Systems International for a quote on the same project. As soon as Bev Morgan heard we had agreed to the project, he scheduled a meeting at our shop.

Bev and Skip Dunham arrived at two o'clock for our appointment. The meeting was short. Bev advised us to cancel our intended proposal and, after a rather heated discussion, we agreed.

When Jim Middleton got wind of this situation, he changed directions by advertising for a bid on twelve new helmets to be designed by the contractor from the bottom up. Writing the standards for this would be very involved, and the lab sent their engineer for scuba training. The complexity of the task was almost too involved for us to comprehend, and their engineer, who had little diving experience and no experience in commercial diving, was soon hopelessly lost.

This was the first time a navy diving helmet would be designed to satisfy the requirements of three separate missions. The underseas tasks began with re-breathers for the SEAL teams; then came the workday demands of the harbor repair divers; and, finally, the spook diving team needed helmets for their then-classified deep saturation assignments on nuclear subs.

Twelve helmets were to be constructed within a thirteen-month time frame. We would be required, by contract, to guarantee satisfaction in all three areas, including the very deep capability involving stringent acceptable flow rates. We were to do all the expensive and complex testing ourselves, and this testing would be verified by the navy lab in Panama City. If the lab determined we had fallen short in any aspect, we would not receive our third and final payment.

Losing this final third would ruin us, so the contract was an invitation to the poorhouse. We would not only have to purchase or rent over $1,000,000 worth of testing equipment, but we would have to make enough money with the first two payments to cover us in case we failed the third.

Scott hired two men to assist me with the bid; my old friend Greg Bryant, an engineer with a mechanical degree, and Doug Smith, a retired navy spook diver. Our study consumed two reams of paper and took us a month to complete. Our bid was $2,500,000, a true value for the navy if there ever was one, and we shipped the proposal on the last hour of the last day.

Our phone rang. Those at the navy lab thought our engineering was excellent and we were told, unofficially, to proceed with the thirteen-month task. The phone rang again the following day. Our bid had exceeded their estimate, for the young navy engineer had expected a bid of just over $1,000,000 which, as I mentioned earlier, was barely enough to pay for the testing equipment rental, much less the costs for design and construction. And even though their man had never been in the manufacturing business, his estimate was considered sacred. We would not be awarded the contract and, because all other bids were subject to the same limitations, the project was dead; a victim of inexperienced engineers at the naval lab.

Scott was beside himself. The upfront money expended on the proposal was down the drain. He phoned Jim Middleton and vented his rage, threatening dire consequences if the navy attempted to use any of our designs in the future. Middleton understood Scott's position but didn't appreciate the way my boss addressed him.

Several months later the navy again advertised for bids. This time it was for a design that was conceived by their young engineer rather than by bidding contractors. When we read the package, it boggled our minds.

As before, the development funds were to be allocated by the same three navy dive groups and included the same penalty. This time, however, the design was to incorporate a removable rear shell to accommodate differing head sizes. This complicated weight-saving plan was required by navy SEALS. They would be wearing hats during a HALO parachute insertion with the diver exiting a high-flying airplane, free-falling for a long distance, and then deploying his chute at minimum altitude. When wearing a normal, heavy, twenty-seven pound helmet, the shock resulting from the parachute opening could put excessive stress on the jumper's neck.

We called their young engineer and suggested lightening the helmet by installing a water-filled rubber bladder to eliminate the design's dead air space and the ballast it required. He would have no part of this change, and we would be required to build the helmets per bid-design. No changes were allowed.

When we noticed the requirement that, after surviving the jump, the diver must have the ability to go to a depth of four hundred feet and remain there for twelve hours, we explained that there was no method in existence that would keep a self-contained diver warm at that depth, and that an adequate gas supply did not exist that would allow him to decompress. I got the same reaction. Don't question why. Just do it.

Our bid was once again completed just under the wire and, after a week had passed, we received a form letter stating that it was unacceptable because of sub-standard engineering. Because the bids from other companies were also unacceptable, the helmets were never built, and I doubt they ever will be. Once again, the men in the naval lab shot holes in their own feet.

After considerable hard work, Scott and our engineering team succeeded in securing a contract from Martin Marietta to design and construct a training arm for NASA. This tool would be used to educate and train the space shuttle team on the use of their new space arm. We soon discovered the space industry might be more messed up than the navy's underseas lab, if such a thing is possible.

Our bid was low even though we had to modify it after being informed the arm was to conform to flight standards, an unnecessary and expensive requirement. The training arm never flew through space, the flight requirements remained, and the arm remained in a room someplace in downtown Houston.

Scott hired Robin Gauss and Brian Macy as our prime engineers. Robin, who had been a commercial diver in the early days of offshore oil, had worked his way through Cal Poly and emerged as a bona fide mechanical engineer while Brian had a degree in agricultural mechanical engineering. I was to work in the capacity of an engineer — an old abalone diver who would be depending upon the talents of others as my sounding board and backup.

By this time Brian, Robin, and other qualified engineers were using the computer for drafting. Recognizing my own shortcomings, I set up an eight-foot-long drafting table and agreed to make a full-size drawing of the arm, then mock it up.

NASA had not required this, but we felt that a mockup was a necessity in order to properly plan the wire loom made up of over a hundred individual wires. This bundle was to run over and around all the arm's joints, and I attacked the project with gusto.

We were under the mistaken impression that Martin Marietta actually wanted a working arm within the deadline and at the bid price. We did not know that Martin had already selected Western Space and Marine because we were considered to be the company most likely to fail. This experienced space firm would then approach Uncle Sam and request a cost overrun. An old trick.

Looking back, it is a wonder we were able to complete the job. From the beginning Robin was the only one who possessed an honest understanding of the task. In order to come up to speed on gear drives, Brian was forced to do a lot of reading. (He was a quick study!) I was a former diver who had taken drafting in high school and depended upon an intuitive understanding of mechanical engineering. And Troy was but four years out of machine school. Our facility was run down, and we did not possess state-of-the-art computers. As a group our chances appeared quite dismal; which was possibly the reason we were hired in the first place.

Kelly Crowcoft, Martin Marietta's in-house design and quality control inspector, was assigned to us, and I'm sure this quiet and reserved man had many doubts. He would walk around, observe us at work, and shake his head. By the end of the job I'm sure he not only liked, but also respected, us.

Our boss, Scott, had one personality flaw. He wanted to do good by everyone. It's my guess that he considered himself to be one of God's helpers, and he never gave up on a person, even if that person was dumb as a stick. Over the years he hired three who fit this "dumb stick" description and, in an attempt to build their self-confidence, he designated each as an "engineer" or "controller." The rest of us were not as kind. "Good grief," someone would remark, "he's doing it again."

But we loved our boss and we always did our best to assist each new "helper." There were a few times when I entertained the thought of eliminating one of them permanently, but then I would change my mind and get drunk at the sports bar across the street.

One individual, Tom, sticks out vividly in my mind. He drove a station wagon filled with an assortment of junk that accumulated day by day until there was barely enough room for him to sit behind the steering wheel. I don't know how he retained his driver's license, for he appeared to be practically blind. The lenses on his glasses were half-an-inch thick and covered with dust and grease. I confiscated them one day and, after cleaning them, he was amazed. "I can see!" he exclaimed. A couple days later, of course, they were dirty again.

Scott, in an effort to assist in our new employee's education, announced that Tom would be doing the wire runs on the arms, and I suggested that it might be better if he worked on something else. "He had extensive training in electronics," Scott informed me, "and he was highly regarded in the Radio Club."

It was apparent that Scott really liked the man or else felt very sorry for him. In either case, we were stuck and we did our best to get along with him. My efforts, alone, entitled me to a place in the Actor's Hall of Fame.

Anyway, Tom fussed around with the wire bundle for months and eventually constructed a single disk of sheet metal which he referred to as the "Cobra Head." This device was supposed to wind up a spool of the umbilical, just behind the end defector where the tools were to be attached. This plan would allow the wire adequate slack; unfortunately, the Cobra Head would have blocked the view of the television camera, rendering the entire arm useless.

Kelly grew uneasy, took me aside, and suggested I take the little bastard to the end of Stearns Wharf and drown him. Then one day, with no particular provocation, I took Tom off the project. "You can't fire me," he exclaimed. "Scott likes me and you need me to wire the arm."

"Bull shit," I told him. "You're fired from the project. If you can see the floor, sweep it!" Then I constructed the necessary hardware and wired the arm as I had intended from the beginning. Kelly, all smiles, took me out to lunch.

The arm was a whopping success, coming in under budget and ahead of schedule. Martin Marietta ran a story in their newsletter claiming "Western Space and Marine is now considered to be our high performance team."

The aerospace firm eventually fired every one of the Martin troops, including Kelly, whom they considered to be responsible for a project that was a success but failed to provide their planned, lucrative, cost overruns.

The aerospace world is an ugly world indeed.

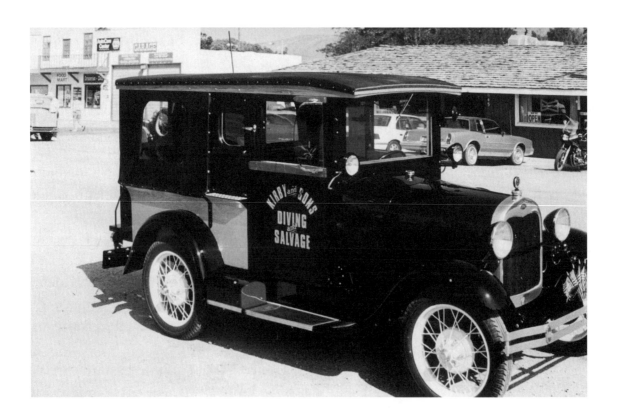

McDONNELL DOUGLAS

Most of the Western Space and Marine employees were great to work with and many became Claudia and my personal friends, particularly Scott and his wife, Carol. Of course there were exceptions.

Remaining true to his compassionate character, Scott hired a third (and last) loser, Fred, an aging Italian whom Scott located through a state employment agency designed to re-educate people with problems. And Lord knows, Fred had problems. I have no idea how he earned his degree in electronic engineering – perhaps he retrieved it from a box of Cracker Jacks – for he didn't know a nut from a bolt or a wire from rope.

Fred spent his days busily plotting colored graphs on his old Mac computer, then running the length of the shop with crumpled papers in his hands and asking stupid questions. He had a habit of grabbing his forehead with both hands and shaking his head from side to side and, just to get rid of him, he was often sent on wild goose chases. He was never sure if we were working on the Martin arm, a cement mixer, or a broken toilet valve.

After we had finished the Martin project, I was assigned to build a positioner for McDonnell Douglas, a device simulating a space walk and designed to align the astronaut with his underwater work stations in a large water tank.

Steve Trotter, a new man assigned to assist me, was a machinist, rigger, and mechanic. He was as good as they come and a pleasure to work with. His jaw had almost been blown away during the war in Viet Nam and it was held together with wire. Though he was in constant pain, he seldom mentioned it. He had an amazing attitude and, working together, we made short work of the rather complex task.

This air-operated, fifteen-foot-long positioner was designed to move ten feet in one direction, four feet in another, and three feet up and down. It would set in a water tank at the McDonnell Douglas plant in Costa Mesa. The ten-foot travel, like that of the other two axis, was driven by a fixed worm gear shaft, one-and-half inches in diameter. Driving on this threaded rod was a rotating nut operated by an air motor and pulling its respective carriage along. Our major problem was that the heavy long shaft was only supported at its ends. It sagged three inches at the center, binding the rotating nut.

My solution was to pre-bend the shaft in the opposite direction, and we accomplished this by placing the ends on wooden blocks and then jumping on the worm. We would re-shim the blocks and repeat the jumping until the bend was exactly what we wanted. When we were finished we called Fred and told him the shaft he had ordered had arrived bent.

"What are you going to do about it?" we asked. He checked the worm that was bent in a rather handsome arc as it lay on the ground.

Just as we expected, he grabbed his head and started to utter, "Mama Mia"; then he yelled, "Mama Mia!!" And he took off, running the entire length of the shop. We never told him we were messing with his head. "What are we going to do today?" someone would ask.

"Oh, I don't know. Let's screw around with Fred."

Suddenly one day, Fred was gone. Thank God for small favors.

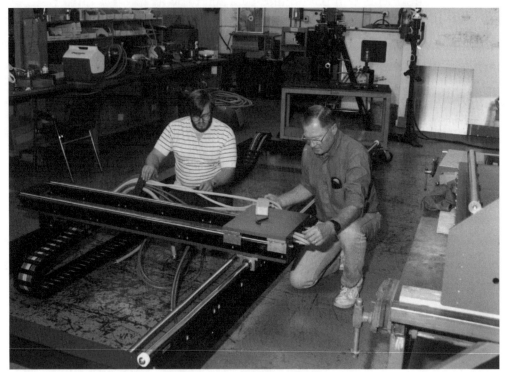

STEVE TROTTER AND BOB

When the positioner was complete, I called Phil Fusion, the McDonnell Douglas man in charge of the program, and he said he would show up the following day for the final evaluation. Scott, who was on a sales trip, had instructed his right hand man, Ben Ortiz, to make sure everything was in place and to videotape the entire transaction.

Tom had remained a thorn in my side, and he talked Ben into allowing his girlfriend to do the videotaping. "She just graduated from Brooks Institute of Photography with a 4.0 GPA," he told Ben. Ben agreed and, nudged by foreboding, I went the sports bar down the street. I had no idea what was in store for us the next day, but I had a feeling it would be disastrous.

Ben showed up at eight the following morning in his business suit and carrying a clipboard, stopwatch, and rule. "Don't worry about a thing," he assured me. "I've been through these evaluation sessions many times. I'll measure everything and make sure it's what Phil Fusion wants."

I wasn't worried about the evaluation session. The sale was a sure thing; I had done my homework. When Phil arrived, all he wished to do was play with the monster.

When Tom and his girlfriend walked in at nine, he was guiding her so she wouldn't bump into things. I took him aside. "You piece of crap," I told him, "your girlfriend is blind."

"Don't worry, Kirby," he assured me. "She got very good grades in school and she'll do a super job."

Steve Trotter and my son Troy set up the rented video camera on its tripod and aimed it in the direction of the action. Then Tom's lady friend pressed the red button down, never letting it up until the battery was dead. Steve inserted another battery while Troy went shopping for a third — a battery with enough life to complete the take of our evaluation, we hoped.

When we played the videotape back, we had two hours of the inventory rack. Our videographer had never moved the camera. Debra, our controller, handed her a rather handsome check for having accomplished absolutely nothing.

When Scott returned to the shop, he was very angry; first at Ben and then at his worthless helper. I considered Scott's outburst to be long overdue.

Scott was often away on sales trips, and he and Ben covered half the states demonstrating a small arm we had just completed. During one of their lengthy absences I decided to clean up our facility, and I hired a young man, Larry, to do some painting. He claimed to be experienced, but I ended up teaching him how to do almost everything. Fortunately, he was trainable and reliable, always showed up on time, and worked hard. He had a great attitude but he had one small hang-up. Though he had never been in the service he appeared enamored with the military and insisted on addressing Steve and me as "sir." As he went about the job, he almost clicked his heels. Steve and I did not enjoy the "sir" crap. We'd both had enough of that.

The remodeling went well; Scott would phone, I would give him a progress report, and he would demand I stop until he arrived back. I never stopped, and we managed to get the place cleaned up before his return, not an easy job because Scott insisted on saving everything. His lifetime collection of junk filled the shop and covered our essential work benches. He never threw anything away, and most of his boxes were covered with mold.

Another time when Scott was out of town I was filling our enormous dumpster when he returned unannounced. Excusing myself by claiming a severe headache, I ran like hell to my car and drove the thirty miles to our home to avoid having both arms broken. He was later seen inside the steel container, tossing out everything I had tossed in.

Oh well, as they say, nobody's perfect. Scott is one of the most loveable men I've ever known, and he runs a very successful engineering firm. Everything he designed not only worked but came in on budget. That's more than can be said for most engineering houses.

I love him, though there were times I could have killed him. And I'm sure there were many times he would have been happy to terminate my freckled frame as well.

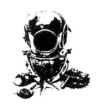

FILMING OF THE *ABYSS*

Scott had been cleaning off his desk, and there were two square-foot clearings now instead of one. The second square-foot section was reserved by Scott for items requiring immediate attention (none of which was ever attended to) while the original section contained his damned telephone. Scott could spend more time on the phone while saying absolutely nothing than anyone I've ever known. Even when a conversation was over, it was impossible to tell him "goodbye" because he refused to hang up.

One day in early spring, 1989, he received a call from Al Giddings, the well-known underwater film maker. Al wanted to reach Bev Morgan, and he had been given the Western Space and Marine number by mistake. When Scott asked what the call regarded, Giddings told him that Twentieth Century Fox needed eleven diving helmets designed and built for *The Abyss*, Jim Cameron's upcoming movie.

My boss quickly took advantage of the situation. "You don't want Bev Morgan," he insisted. "You want Bob Kirby, and he works for me." Scott can be very persuasive, and Giddings forgot all about Bev.

Scott and I drove down to the Century City studio and, when Jim Cameron and I met, we immediately liked one another. During the next year and a half, my feelings for this outstanding director never diminished. I understand that some consider him to be an ill-tempered tyrant, quick to order people off the set, but I seldom saw him in this light. Though he was, admittedly, all work and no play, he also had a sense of humor, and I was privileged to enjoy this side of his personality. By the time the production of *The Abyss*, came to an end — a film that is considered to be one of the "toughest shoots in history" — we were good friends and we remain so today.

Scott and I watched Ron Cobb, the talented artist whose loose renderings would guide the film, sketch the helmets. Could we build them as they had been drawn and still make them work? I was sure we could.

Back at our shop, Scott and I worked up a design-bid which included eleven helmets and backpacks; ten for the actors and one for Cameron who would be wearing his while directing the underwater sequences. His hat had to work, and it had to work well.

Because no umbilicals were to be used, all breathing air had to be supplied by the backpacks; consequently, free-flow helmets would be far too wasteful. We had to create a design faithful to Ron's drawings, displaying a full view of the actor's faces while incorporating a demand-breathing system without oral nasal masks. While I was assuring him I could do this, I crossed my fingers behind my back. I had no idea how to accomplish it without killing an actor or two with carbon dioxide buildup.

The hats also had to be outfitted with phones allowing hard wires to topside as the need arose; another bucketful of snakes.

There were other challenges. We were to build an underwater, high-pressure air manifold with whips so four divers could simultaneously fill their air backpacks on the bottom. This scheme was required so that the first actors on the set could top off their air supplies just before the last members of the filming crew were in place, a generally time-consuming process.

Cameron had a final requirement; he wanted us to furnish a man to tend to his personal underwater needs and maintain the other ten rigs for the entire length of the underwater filming. This would take approximately a year.

After many hours of hard thinking and pencil work, Scott sent them a bid covering everything for $300,000. The ensuing silence was deafening, and Scott eventually followed up with a phone call. He came into the shop, crumbled FAX in hand, and reported their reply. They would build the helmets themselves before they would spend $300,000.

"Okay, Scott," I said. "Give them a bid they can't refuse. Make it $62,500." He looked at me as if I had lost it. "There's no way we can do the job for that!" he insisted.

"Trust me, Scott," I said. "Just make the call."

When he returned he looked relieved as well as perplexed. "Okay," he said, "they jumped at the price. The project is ours. I just hope we don't end up in the poorhouse."

Several days later I asked Scott to call Cameron's office and see if they wanted communications in the hats for an extra $20,000, as the base price didn't include these. They didn't flinch.

A couple of weeks later I advised Scott to ask Fox if they wanted the backpacks to supply batteries for the helmet's lights. "Hell yes," was the answer. I followed this up with questions regarding buoyancy control, manuals, and training. By the time they were nearing completion of the movie, our total invoices totalled close to $300,000. We could live with that and, now, so could Fox.

We settled on a servo-demand system for the helmets, an approach that had never succeeded before. But I felt confident we could overcome the many obstacles and make the design work. And it did...well...kind of. Unfortunately, it was extremely unpleasant to use.

Without an oral nasal mask, one of Ron Cobb's requirements, the air had to blow in with strong force and volume in order to clear the excessive carbon dioxide buildup. This onslaught of air over-pressured the hat's interior, shutting off the servo airflow. As the diver continued to inhale, the cycle repeated itself three times and the diver's head was shaken in the process.

I was wrong to expect I could dampen the system with pneumatic tricks and snake oil. Experiments, time, and money were the only things that could completely take care of our problems, and we had none of these as both our due date and our funding were tight as hell.

All *The Abyss* hats were somewhat uncomfortable, depending upon the view. By the end of the year Cameron hated his blue helmet with the white star on each side, and I'm sure he spent many evenings poking pins into my voodoo doll. He would show me the sore spots under his chin and grumble; at the same time, he understood our dilemma. Well...perhaps. I would listen sympathetically, then go after coffee for both of us, chuckling along the way. I knew the whole story, and I also knew enough to keep it to myself. Just as it had been with Bev and me and the Sea Lab helmets, there had been no funding for research and development. And, as we might have expected, the end result was turning into a nighttime duck shoot with no moon.

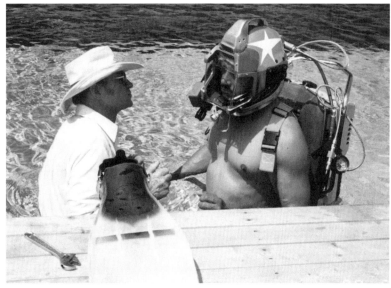

BOB ORIENTING JIM CAMERON IN HIS STAR HELMET
GAFFNEY, SOUTH CAROLINA

Looking back, I am amazed at what we had accomplished. I doubt Jim Cameron shared my jubilation; the low price being much sweeter than the product.

We had five months in which to complete and deliver the systems. I made a time-line chart, and we lived by it. When we fell behind I worked weekends to make up the lost time. Robin Gauss designed and built the backpacks, my son Troy designed and machined the regulators, and I made the patterns for the brass castings. I ordered all the castings at once, not knowing if they would work or not — a long shot that paid off. I also designed and built the molds for the helmets.

We located a fiberglass movie firm in the Los Angeles area; Don Penington made the backpacks and helmet shells here which saved us a lot of time. Don was another splendid man, eager and honest.

I rehired Larry Smith who had assisted me during the facelift of Scott's shop. He was one of the most reliable men I've ever known, and he eventually accompanied us to Long Beach, California, to assist with the shoot. At first everyone got along with Larry, but his conservative political views were not appreciated by the more liberal actors and occasionally things turned very vocal. However, though I sometimes wanted to shut him up, I don't know what I would have done without him.

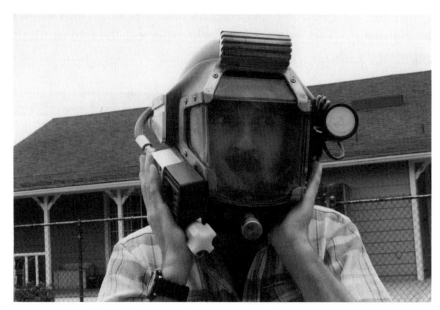

JIM CAMERON IN OUR FIRST PROTOTYPE AT MY HOME

Six weeks after hiring Larry our first helmet was ready for in-water testing. I shaved material from the heavy upper handle that doubled as a weight until the hat balanced under water. Then I constructed a new handle pattern and ordered thirteen castings.

One day Jim Cameron showed up at the pool where I had made history with the invention of the yoke retention system and air hat Bev and I had sold to the navy some fifteen years earlier. He was not interested in my past, my shop, or our house. A very focused individual, he was there to videotape the hat underwater and mandate any changes necessary; not to join a social club. I spent the day as an actor, making faces and swimming around for his camera, and he drove away pleased with his underwater footage.

Keeping up with our schedule grew more and more difficult; the harder we worked, the behinder we got. I had to write an operation's manual for our gear before we were to leave for Gaffney, South Carolina, and I decided to make it pictorial. I completed it in two days — one day before our departure.

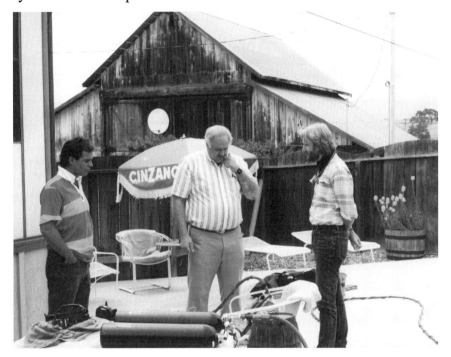

SCOTT MILLARD, JIM CAMERON, SANTA YNEZ CALIFORNIA

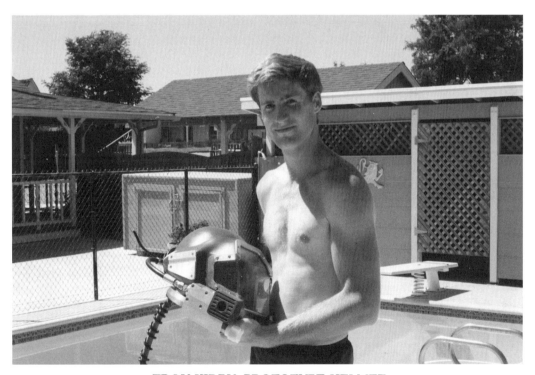

TROY KIRBY, PROTOTYPE HELMET

Scott insisted we test the helmets and backpacks before shipping them to the unfinished nuclear generating plant in Gaffney and, just as we feared, we ran out of time. I knew Cameron well enough to not ask for more time; a simple "I'm working on it," was far more positive.

The first time a helmet and backpack were together underwater was on the body of leading actor Ed Harris and, as I had suspected, he knew little about the workings of diving helmets. By the time he surfaced, as his instructor, the beads of sweat on my forehead were as large as horse turds.

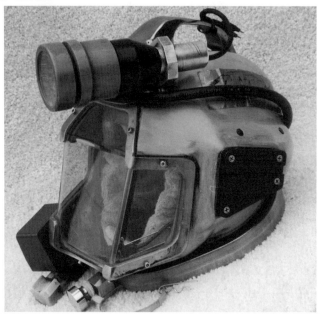

ONE OF THE WESTERN SPACE AND MARINE *ABYSS* HELMETS, 1990

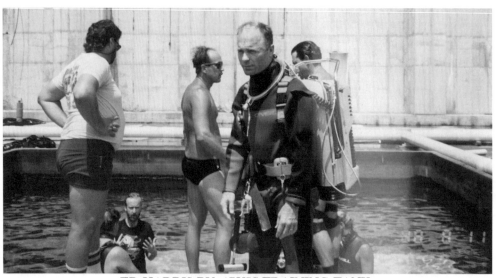

ED HARRIS BY *ABYSS* TRAINING TANK

Ed was a number-one athlete and a hell of a man, and I really appreciated him. He was also the only guy on the set who could challenge Jim Cameron and get away with it.

Al Giddings, Scott and I gave splendid directions to everyone involved, stressing the layers of safety to be employed during all shoots. Our concerns were acknowledged and the actors, exposed only to the basics of scuba at a topless facility in the Caribbean, became anxious. In fact, they were scared as hell.

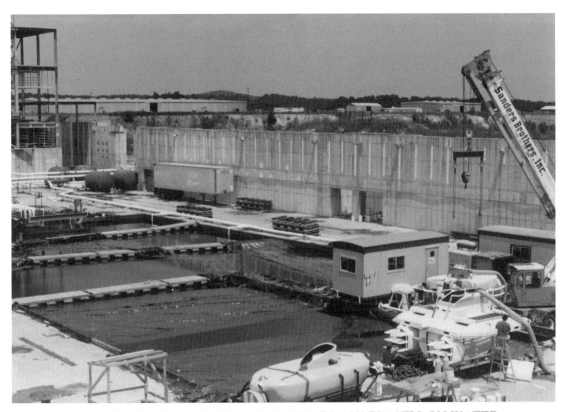

SHALLOW TANK, CAB ONE, FLATBED, BLACK PLASTIC ON WATER

I dressed into a rig and descended twenty-five feet to the bottom of a huge, rectangular, black, gunite-lined concrete tank while Cameron followed, filming me as I ran up the walls and did flips. The actors at the "dailys" viewed the footage at the end of each day and, once they were assured the rigs worked, it was up to them – and me – to work out any problems involving the gear or the actors wearing it. Both were tough calls.

One important detail was the matter of clearing the actors' ears, something Cameron had felt unnecessary while the helmets were being designed. (Perhaps he had figured, since actors can walk on water, their ears wouldn't need clearing.) I installed pads for them to place their beaks against and blow; a throwback to my old abalone days.

The sixty-feet deep, two-hundred-foot-diameter, uncompleted, nuclear plant tank was originally intended to house a nuclear reactor. In the event of a meltdown, two eight-foot-diameter penstocks were to be opened, flooding the tank with water from an adjacent lake. Water from this lake had been used to fill one of the other, smaller tanks which we were using for training. Once in a while a water moccasin would find its way into this tank, resulting in chaos. I hate snakes and Claudia, always nearby, freaked out.

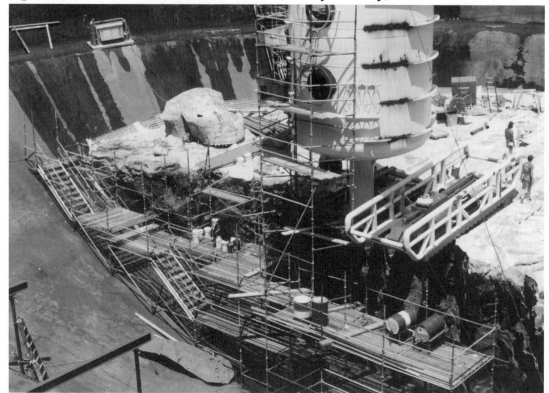

MAIN SET, ROUND TANK, 200' x 60' DEEP

To overcome the severe problem with green algae, generated by the humid South Carolina weather, enormous filters were installed and two dump trucks filled with dry chlorine were added. Very soon, our colorful bathing suits were shades of mottled gray with splotches of white, our hair was green, and our skins burned like hell. Because so much chlorine was being used, the large steel underwater movie props began to rust, plugging the filtering system and turning the once crystal-clear water to a putrid brown. The company in charge of servicing the filters, not anticipating the filters reaction to so much chlorine, had taken several days off.

Cameron began to chew ass and, when he had finished chewing, he fired his assistant director. Meanwhile, I cleaned the filters and we were back in business. There was one silver lining to the chlorine situation; the water moccasins died.

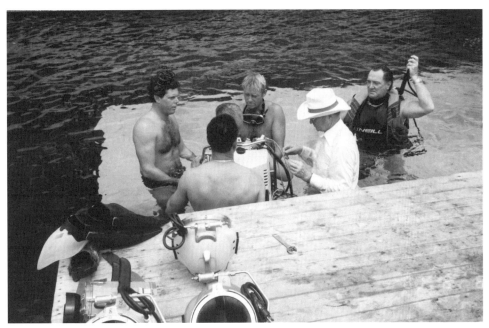

TRAINING TANK, KIRBY IN WHITE HAT, AL GIDDINGS BEHIND KIRBY

I worked closely with Al Giddings and his crew and with Jim Cameron. Al told me he never hired a diver if the individual did not have a trade. "We don't hire divers," he said. "They are a dime a dozen. I need electricians, carpenters, machinists, and photographic experts." I liked Giddings. He was a bright guy and a fine man.

Two large vans held everything Al and his crew might need, including a small machine shop. I particularly appreciated the machine shop because by the time shooting began, Gaffney was a sauna. As a result of the extreme heat, the servo-demand valves began to seize. Using Al's lathe, I was able to machine down their sliding pistons, thereby saving the day. Hell, the entire shoot.

As I said, Giddings and his men were as good as they come; actually, so was everyone else on the set. I've never been in the company of so many talented individuals. Everyone was helpful and courteous, no matter how many hours we worked each day; and fourteen hours seemed to be the average.

Claudia and I, as the oldest people on the set, were the most impacted. Fortunately, Cameron liked "older folks" and made concessions for our age. The younger people were not as lucky, and when Troy joined us Jim gave him as hard a time as I had expected.

Claudia stayed with me for the five weeks we were in South Carolina, and she worked as hard as anyone, but without pay. My petite wife cleaned the sets, raked the pot-holed pavement, and attempted to "make things nice." Cameron, not missing a thing, included her in the film's credits as "Best Girl," a title she earned by using a rake, not by "servicing" the troops as one gaffer had jokingly suggested.

241

When Cameron saw the helmets and backpacks for the first time, he gave me a direct order to "mess them up." The original contract had mandated they look old and well-used but Scott, who was extremely proud of the gear, had ignored the order and they arrived on the set in perfect condition.

One day Claudia and I were tasked to paint some of the helmets, and to do this quickly. I ran to the paint locker, cleaned a spray gun belonging to the film company's painter, and shot the hats. (Using a spray gun belonging to another person is akin to sleeping with someone else's wife and, after I was through, the painter entered the shop. I felt as if I'd been caught with my hands in the cookie jar, but when he noticed I had cleaned the gun after using it, he smiled and told me I was welcome to help myself anytime.)

Anyway, Cameron showed up in paint locker where Claudia and I were hard at work. "Goddamn it, Bob," he yelled. "I want them to look frigging OLD! Here, give me one." He took a helmet and began to scrape it over the rough concrete floor. The floor had been repainted several times, and the deep scratches Cameron was putting in the helmet picked up the many colors. The helmet eventually resembled the bottom of a beached sailing ship on a coral reef.

I started on the other hats, and then the backpacks received the same loving care. Using a large brush, I painted everything with black lacquer. After wiping most of the lacquer off, the helmets appeared to be covered in dried oil. The large WSM logos on the backpacks were almost destroyed in the process.

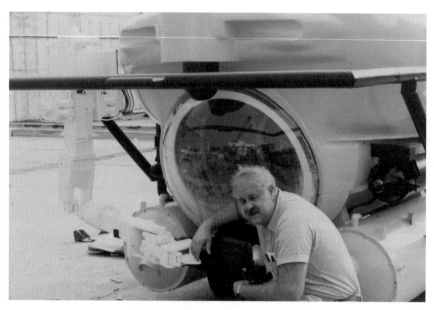

SCOTT MILLARD, CAB ONE

When Scott entered the paint locker to see if he could help, he almost cried. "Oh, Bob," he wailed, "my beautiful helmets...all messed up. Couldn't you have done something else?" I told him that Cameron had done the scraping; I had just followed suit.

We had lots of fun that day!

A pecking order is observed during the production of a film, and Wardrobe is near the top of the list. Deborah Everton was in charge of Wardrobe for the filming of *The Abyss* and she made sure everyone knew it. Her temper was as hot and humid as the interior of her trailer, a structure with genuine wooden steps that had been constructed for her by a carpenter on the set.

To access the trailer occupied by Western Space and Marine, we had to climb a pile of awkward and dangerous pallets. Scott decided we needed the steps leading to Wardrobe, and he dragged them to our trailer. Deborah and her troops would no longer be able to safely exit Wardrobe; that large step to the ground was a mother!

Claudia ran to the rescue, and the words she and Scott exchanged punctured the humid air as they stood on opposite ends of the stairs and pulled. My wife eventually won the tug-of-war, an act of kindness that possibly saved us from being forcibly evicted from the set. Helmets or no helmets, I'm sure we would have been on the next plane west.

The film's story line portrays an enormous, combined, underwater saturation system, an oil-drilling rig beneath a thousand feet of water. In order to create the illusion of depth and darkness, truckloads of black phenolic beads were dumped onto the surface of the water, eliminating all light. The actors, already less than enthusiastic about diving, were to descend to the tank floor, then make their way in total darkness – perhaps two hundred feet to the set – with Al Gidding's safety divers assisting.

Accomplishing this in total darkness was understandably spooky for anyone but a seasoned diver; thank God Jim Cameron chose a bona fide commercial diver, Captain Kid Brewer, Jr., as one of his actors, for Kid assisted the others through the ordeal. I doubt whether the film would have been successful without him. Many of the scenes were just too tough for fledgling divers unfamiliar with commercial diving equipment, and I'm convinced some accidents would have resulted.

One accident that was nearly fatal took place on the morning of what was to be Claudia and my last day on the South Carolina set. As a result of my lifting the seventy-pound backpacks, my shoulders had been troubling me, and I needed a doctor to look at them. Scott had long since returned to Santa Barbara, and my son Troy had been sent to replace me.

In the movie, Leo Burmester portrayed the character Catfish; he was well-cast as the burly, underwater roughneck. A soft-spoken man, he was also adept at dealing with ongoing problems on the set. I had no idea Leo also possessed a temper.

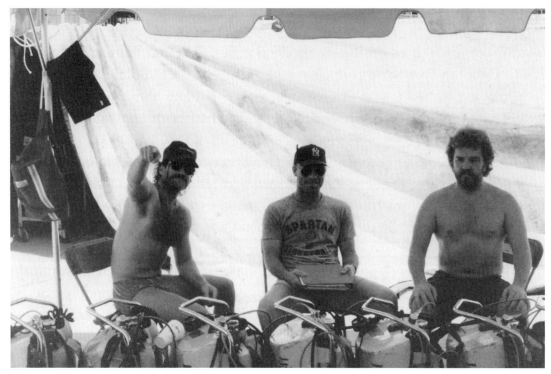

L to R: CAPTAIN KIDD BREWER, ED HARRIS, LEO BURMESTER

Troy and I were dressing in the actors for a take that involved the five of them on the bottom at one time, and Leo was the last to don his diving helmet. Usually very easy to get along with, Leo appeared to be in a bad mood. I wrestled with him as I placed the helmet over his head and, before I could engage the safety pin, he pushed me aside, slid off the wooden stage and under the black surface to the twenty-five-foot-deep bottom.

Without waiting for one of Al's troops to assist, he took off in a flash, heading into the darkness without knowing which way he was going. I kept my ears open to the microphone hooked into Cameron's hat, even though I was helpless to assist in the event a problem arose.

According to a later report by Al's safety divers, when Leo finally located the set he seemed possessed and was twisting this way and that, pulling on his helmet's neck ring latch in an apparent effort to attain more comfort. As he made it to his location, high on the set, he continued to jerk on his helmet.

Then I heard Cameron's words over the speaker. "A diver is in trouble." Leo's hat had come off and, filled with water, it was now a twenty-five-pound anchor pulling him off the set and fifteen feet down to the floor of the tank. Two of the safety divers who came to his aid had attempted to place a demand regulator in his mouth. They were unsuccessful until one held Leo's hands behind him while the other inserted the octopus regulator into his mouth and pressed the purge button.

By the time Leo and the safety diver made their way back to my stage, he had still not completely regained his composure. His helmet hung by its hose and Leo's eyes — red, fiery beads in their deep sockets — bore an expression of deep rage. As a rule, I'm usually able to subdue a person who becomes illogical during a dive, but not Leo. He wanted my blood and, using language I'd never even heard during my four years in the navy, he let me know it.

Once a shooting is underway, a considerable amount of money has been spent on the footage and the plot. If an important actor is suddenly absent from the set, a financial disaster can result. Any person, even the director, who causes an actor to miss a take can be instantly fired. Understanding this, there was no way I could retaliate. I could only run like hell, and I was prepared to do just that.

A stunt man whom I had befriended was standing behind us, and he suddenly leaped over me, took Leo by the shoulders, and spoke softly in his ear. I have no idea what he said but it certainly worked, for Leo settled down, then apologized. We never had another problem with him or with one another. A wonderful actor; his portrayal of Catfish was outstanding.

There is a scene in *The Abyss* where the oil divers encounter the bodies of dead sailors inside a sunken nuclear submarine. The stunt men portraying the corpses had to hyperventilate from hookah rigs for several minutes on pure oxygen, slide the regulators out of sight, hold their breaths, and play dead as the camera panned them.

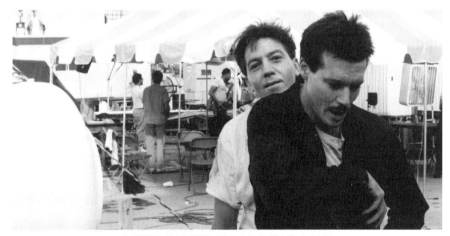

MIKE CAMERON AS DEAD MAN

245

The key stunt man for this take was Jim Cameron's brother, Mike Cameron. Adding drama, Mike Cameron was to hold a small live crab in his mouth. As the camera approached, he opened his mouth on cue to allow the crab to escape. Instead, the crab seized Mike's tongue with his claws and wouldn't let go. In the finished movie, you can see Mike's placid face, then his eyes; alive with anguish as he attempts to break the crab's painful grip.

The character, Jammer, was to be triggered by an oxygen hit at the sight of the dead sailors, and Cameron approached during a lunch break. "What does oxygen poisoning look like?" he asked me. I remembered being inside a chamber with another navy diver and witnessing such an attack.

"It's just like an epileptic fit," I told him. "The diver's eyes roll back and he begins to convulse. Soon his body is bent up and he just quivers." With this I got down on the cement floor and proceeded to demonstrate a seizure.

When I looked up I was surrounded by several actors who had arrived too late to hear our conversation. They were apparently impressed by my talent for improvisation, though it sure cut into their appetites for lunch.

As the film proceeded, the actors became capable divers. I was particularly impressed by their bottom times, because some could stay down over two hours without refilling. They had learned to pace their breathing, and I patted myself on the back. What a good instructor I had been!

I got my comeuppance sometime later when I noticed a massive upheaval of bubbles on the surface of the water, just over the underwater refilling manifold. When I pulled the contraption up, I found air escaping from every valve. Tying it off, I inspected the high-pressure air compressor. Its gauge indicated 4500 pounds. The relief valve had been twisted in, allowing the pressure to far exceed the 3000-pound scuba tank rating. Our actors had almost become swimming bombs. A quick FAX to Santa Barbara and new valves were on the way. I don't believe Cameron or the actors involved ever heard about this possibly fatal situation. If they had known they probably would have conducted an evening ceremony by hanging my freckled nude body out for the no-see-ums to gnaw, for I was the person responsible for inspecting the air compressor each day.

Gaffney was a laid-back southern town with a church on every corner. To celebrate their main industry, summer crops of peaches, the city fathers had replaced the town's old water tank tower with one that was larger and spherical. As with a peach, the tower had a single, giant crease pointing upwards at a forty-five-degree angle. Painted peach-pink, the tower placed Gaffney on the map and into the *Guinness Book of World Records*. One couldn't help noticing, however, that the tower also resembled the bare bottom of an overweight woman, bending over.

To remedy this embarrassing blunder, the city fathers ordered the addition of a peach stem. Now the tower looked like the same fat lady, but with a peach stem protruding from her rectum.

By the end of the long days we were beat, and I was in need of a good drink before our dinner of deep-fried critters (which appeared to be the only meal available in Gaffney). A pleasant, young black lady stood behind the counter of a large grocery store passing items over the electronic counter.

"Excuse me, Ma'am," I said, "where can I buy a bottle of Scotch?"

Without hesitation or even looking up, she said, "Y'all new here in Gaffney, ain't ya?"

"Yes, ma'am, I am."

"Here in Gaffney," she continued, "we's decent folks. If y'all insist on being part of the devil, the state store is in that building just over there with the red ball over the door."

"Oh, great, I can walk to it."

"Oh no you cain't. Y'all have to drive. We needs to know where the likes of y'all are and what kind of car you have."

"You want a bottle of Scotch?" a man now appearing behind the counter said. "May God have mercy on your soul."

As a rule we had breakfast on the set; egg enchiladas and coffee. At this time we outlined the day's activities and organized the troops. One morning at breakfast we observed two seasoned combat-soldier-types wearing dirty khakis, long-ago polished boots, and covered with tatoos. They looked like hell and smelled just as bad, as if they'd been camping for a month. You could tell, by their red faces and veins protruding from their sooted necks, they were very angry.

"Where the hell is Jim Cameron?" one asked. I smiled, then asked them to join us for breakfast and tell us what was wrong.

"What's frigging wrong? The goddammed young kids we're supposed to train are awful bastards. We took them on a two-day bivouac to train them in the ways of fighting men. We had them in a culvert for the evening, eating snakes, bugs, and things like that. Then we tossed in cherry bombs to add a little effect, you know, get real. The next thing we knew, the goddamned kids were gone. The little piss-ants had taken the lake owner's yacht, and they ran to the other side where they beached it. Then the little assholes flanked us and tossed half-sticks of dynamite on top of us. We ended up in the same frigging

247

culvert as they were, and for the whole damned night. Each time we tried to escape, the little bastards would toss in more damned cherry bombs, and from each end. We spent the entire evening in mud filled with frigging snakes and bugs. When Cameron gets here we intend to give him a piece of our minds."

While pretending to share their concerns, I was laughing inside. And when Cameron heard what they had to say, I detected a faint smile as well. Jim had hired these men to instruct the two young actors in combat warfare and they had, obviously, accomplished this mission. Their wards had become seasoned, fighting men. The last we saw of the two combat troops were the backs of their dirty, pointed heads. Cameron was a happy man. The young actors would play their parts well.

In the story line for the film, *The Abyss*, Bud Brigman, as played by actor Ed Harris, drops down the wall of the Cayman Trough to diffuse a nuclear bomb on the Abyssal Plain, two-and-a-half miles below. To accomplish this long descent, the screenwriter supplied Bud with a futuristic "fluid-breathing system" delivering an "oxygenated fluorocarbon emulsion." Actual experiments in liquid breathing have progressed in real laboratories where an anesthetized human volunteer has successfully oxygenated his blood in one fluid-filled lung just as our stunt rat, Beanie, did. The barrier to further progress lies in the fact that lungs (in the rats as well as ours) are just not strong enough to pump fluid comfortably. Also, the water will flush out all the natural bacteria, leaving the survivor to perish from a lung infection. Beanie, however, lived to squeak about it, for he was a tough little critter. Mike Cameron eventually took Beanie home as a pet, but the little rodent, apparently remembering his ordeal, bit the hell out of his new master. (As I write this, an advocate group has probably been formed to lobby for laws against drowning, then reviving, white rats.)

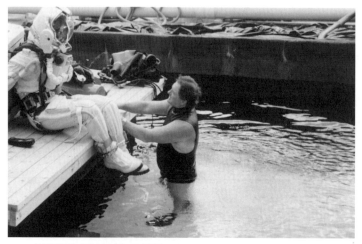

FLUID-FILLED SUIT, AL GIDDINGS IN WATER

248

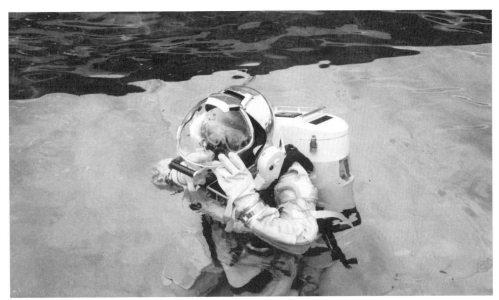

OXYGENATED FLUID-FILLED HELMET DURING TESTS

While I was training the actors, a fine-looking man (whom I never got to know) was tasked with building the liquid-breathing gear. He constructed it with glue, paper, and balsa wood and, though it was fake, it looked very impressive. To create an underwater illusion the prop was designed to be used and filmed in a smoke-filled room. When it arrived in Gaffney, Cameron, apparently forgetting his original instructions, ordered it into the square water tank where one of Gidding's stunt divers hyperventilated from a hookah rig, and then held his breath during the brief test takes.

The apparatus came apart very quickly, and only the fiberglass dome and plexiglass view port survived. The artist and craftsman who built it received a chewing out followed by a plane ticket home.

Wardrobe piled the prop in a heap in its trailer, awaiting someone who could glue it back together. (Perhaps it would jump back together by itself...a bit of Hollywood magic.) Cameron, with so many things on his mind and forgetting about the prop's demise in Gaffney, called. He needed it on the set in Long Beach. Deborah pleaded with me. Could I repair it? She had to have it, and *soon;* before Cameron discovered she had overlooked it.

She coaxed Mike Cameron into heading up the effort, and he arrived at our Western Space and Marine facility in Santa Barbara with what was left of the silver and white rig now crammed inside a large cardboard box.

"Jim wants this rebuilt so it can survive diving," he said, "and he needs it in a week."

"Okay, Mike," I told him. "I'll do my best." (Never say no to James Cameron.)

The only portions of the helmet that would hold up under water were the fiberglass helmet shell and its domed view port, which meant a difficult task lay ahead. Fortunately,

249

Mike stuck around to assist, and he was a particularly competent hand.

Scott phoned Oceaneering and persuaded them to sell Twentieth Century Fox the metal neck ring components for a Rat Hat. According to Ron Cobb's original drawings, these would work well. Now we had to fabricate the metal port frame and modify the fiberglass shell to receive both it and the Rat Hat neck-ring assembly. My shop was better suited than Scott's machine shop for the dirty soldering and grinding metal work involved and, after five long days in my barn, Mike and I could pat ourselves on our backs. The metal components, plated with soft solder to look like dull chrome, turned out well. The fiberglass shell, which we painted a smooth white, also looked very good.

It was time to work on my "gag," which is movie talk for an illusion. In this case the take was of the liquid pouring out of the helmet when Bud removes it after the dive. I machined an O-ring-sealed plug that, outwardly, matched one of the swivels from the helmet to the back pack, and I fitted a rubber, one-way valve inside it. Next we prepared a one-inch hose with a fitting to mate to the plug and a ball valve on the hose's end. The other end of the hose ran to a big bucket of water on top of a ladder.

After Mike put on the helmet and locked the cams down to his neck dam ring, I shoved the hose fitting into the helmet and opened the ball valve. The helmet filled within a couple of seconds while Mike held his breath, and I then removed the fitting.

We videotaped the gag and it went well. Not only was Mike a great stunt man, he was also a good actor. He could hold his breath for a very long time, as the script described; and with a wild look in his eyes. When he released the locking cams and removed the helmet, water poured out. This was exactly the way it was supposed to happen when Bud returned from his deep visit with the frightening underwater creatures that were covered with glowing lights.

Mike drove the videotape down to Long Beach for his brother to view; one week to the day we were ready to film.

The day I was to perform my gag, Claudia and I made our first trip to the Long Beach facility, an enormous WWII vintage seaplane hanger slated to be demolished. Running water, electricity, and sanitary facilities were in poor repair, and power to the hanger's many antique outlets was supplied by huge generators. We had been allotted a small shop in which to house our helmets and the liquid breathing system. This was a blessing as the diving gear required constant maintenance.

A rectangular water tank had been constructed for Cameron. It was fifteen feet high, twenty feet wide, and fifty feet long, with one end constructed of five-inch-thick plexiglass. The hanger floor was the bottom, and the tank's walls were attached to it with anchor bolts and gaskets. Cameron would be filming the liquid breathing descent; many water critters, manipulated by puppeteers on the surface, would also be swimming here.

(We referred to these spooky creations as "the little people.")

I was ordered to ready my gag on the sound stage, and Cameron arrived soon after finishing at another location. The gag came off as well with Ed Harris as it had with Mike; and Robin Oliver, the assistant director, complimented me.

The next gag, a simulation of Ed throwing up water from his lungs, was no small endeavor if it were to appear real. This was the job of our new special-effects team, for Cameron had released Joe Unsinn and his crew after production in Gaffney was completed. The new team was owned by Joe Gaberelli and this was their first day on the set. It was also their first major film.

Because he knew of Cameron's reputation, Gaberelli was as nervous as a long-tailed cat in a room filled with rocking chairs; one screw-up and he and his organization would be history. He wouldn't be able to get a job making bagels. On the other hand, if he survived for the balance of the film, he would have made a name for himself.

Ed Harris was on his knees and a small hose running from a Hudson weed sprayer was taped to his left cheek and terminated alongside his mouth, out of camera view. "Okay, Ed," Cameron yelled. (Actual sound is dubbed later so loud instructions like these can be safely issued.)

Ed convulsed realistically, but the puny stream of water leaving his mouth, not unlike a boy peeing, was not convincing. "Cut it!" Cameron shouted. "Goddamn it Joe! What kind of crap is this?! Do you think you can talk Bob Kirby into letting us use his frigging bucket and hose?"

By combining my one-inch hose and fluid convincingly colored with cranberry juice, the gag was a big success. For the time being, Joe and his crew were still on board; Cameron might even have felt a bit sorry for them. However, everyone knew that, one more screw-up, Joe and his crew would be history. And even though I had saved his ass, Joe now disliked me with a vengeance.

In the next scene, to be shot in the rectangular tank, Bud — wearing the liquid-filled diving equipment — appeared to be falling down the wall of the abyss. Mike Cameron and I had our act together; the gear was ready and the take would be a piece of cake if the filming crew didn't blow their end.

Al Giddings and his film crew had not been invited to Long Beach. Instead, Cameron had hired his old friend Michael Salomon, to do the filming. The reflectors and lighting were to be held in place by divers from Joe's new team, and everyone was anxious to see them in action.

Deborah of Wardrobe had a sharp eye, and she directed my attention to a perplexed looking Joe, sitting alone on the upper edge of the tank with his rented scuba gear while his divers were at their assignments inside the tank. "Is it my imagination," she asked me, "or does Joe not know a thing about diving?"

I observed Joe studying his rig. "Debbie," I said, "I think you're right. Don't worry, I'll see what I can do."

As good fortune would have it, Cameron and Ed Harris had not yet arrived on the set so I had some time. I sat down by the special-effects man who was not terribly pleased to see me. "Joe," I said, "you don't know anything about what you're holding, do you?" He admitted he did not. "Okay," I continued, "let's just pretend we're talking about sex or politics. I'll act as if I'm looking around the hanger while you keep your eyes on the rig and I'll tell you about it." He didn't say a word.

"It's my guess you learned to dive in the 50s and 60s, long before this rig was invented. Is that correct? He nodded and I continued. "This rig has two demand regulators instead of one. That thing in your hand is called an octopus. Its purpose is to be capable of supplying air to another diver in an emergency. Got that?" He continued to nod. "The bag and extra mouthpiece on a hose is the buoyancy compensator, or BC. If you lift the hose and squeeze the button, air will come out and you will sink. The bag can be inflated by either blowing into the mouthpiece on the hose or by pressing the other button to power-inflate the bag. That's all there is to it."

Joe looked at the rig for a moment, I helped him don it, and then he slipped under the surface where he assisted in setting up the many lights and reflectors. We remained friends for the rest of the project and, as far as I know, Cameron kept him on board.

On our last day at the Long Beach facility, Cameron was to be underwater during the filming of the final shots of Bud who was now being portrayed by stunt man, Charlie Arneson. Charlie, who would be falling the two-and-a-half miles down the wall, was able to hold his breath longer than anyone I had ever known. I fed him oxygen for five minutes, then he put his regulator in his mouth and descended to his mark. He removed the regulator, closed the plexiglass port, and held his breath while the cameras rolled.

For this episode, Ed Harris was used only when the camera showed his face. Considering he was inexperienced as a diver and the fact that he was a smoker, he did a remarkable job. I have no idea how he could hold his breath as long as he did without turning blue.

Knowing Cameron was scheduled to be on the underwater set in half an hour, I grabbed his hat and ran. I could not get over how light it was and had gone fifty feet when I realized the neck ring assembly was still on the bench. Because of a failed glue joint, it had broken clearly away. I thanked God this had happened when it did, for if it had failed underwater, we would have had a serious problem on our hands.

Running back to the facility, I ground both surfaces and, using auto body filler, I reglued the ring. Mike Cameron had observed the episode, and we made a pact never to tell his brother.

After we moved to the Los Angeles Coliseum to use its large swimming pools to film the scenes containing underwater miniatures, I let Cameron know we had experienced a severe problem with his hat in Long Beach. "Jim," I said, "it was so bad it might have killed you, but I can't tell you what took place."

"Oh sure, Bob," he replied casually, "probably a failed regulator."

"Far worse than that," I told him. "Mike and I each cut a finger, passed blood, and swore one another to secrecy. We can't tell you what happened, and we never will." By now Mike was rolling with laughter. It was hard to get the best of Jim Cameron.

Eleven years later I broke the pact I had made with Mike by explaining what had actually happened. "Jim," I told him, "you would have died. Even worse, Mike and I would have been tasked to complete your film. How's that for a shitty situation!?"

"You know what?" Jim said. "You're an asshole."

"I know," I answered. "I know."

The Coliseum is located in the very bowels of Los Angeles. The sound of gunshots is a constant chorus, sirens wail all through the night, and muggers lurk right outside the locked fence. Our security guard warned us not to venture beyond the gate unless it was a life and death emergency, and he warned us it would very likely be death if we ignored his warning. And he wasn't kidding. Police choppers flew overhead day and night, their blades thump thump thumping and, in the evening when they aimed their spotlights down, they were bright enough to light up an entire city block.

According to *The Abyss* story line, the navy nuclear sub hits the wall of the Cayman Trough and sinks. In preparation for the sinking and resulting crash, Cameron had personally jigsawed the bow of the fifteen-foot model sub so that it would implode convincingly. When it came to getting his hands dirty, he was no slouch; after all, he got his start in the business as a model maker.

Several special-effect troops held a long pole attached to the stern of the model sub and, on cue, they were to shove down on the pole, impacting the model's thin, fiberglass hull against a rock. As it broke apart, tiny pieces of equipment, people, torpedoes, etc. were rigged to fall out. Cameron wasn't satisfied with this scene, and we had to do it a second time which meant recovering everything now lying at the bottom of the pool. Cameron joined us, helped put the pieces back together, and assisted in regluing the hull.

The first time we attempted this take the water was too clear; the second time, the troops on the pole did not push down hard enough and the hull refused to break open; the third time, in order to make the water more obscure, we emptied milk into it. By now the men manning the pole had a thorough understanding of their duties and were ready. Nothing could go wrong for if it did, Cameron would have to repair the sub and no one wanted to be around when that took place.

Our director possessed a remarkable collection of words; most were far stronger than any I wish to print so allow me to paraphrase: "Okay...God damn it...put in the frigging milk...what the hell..it's frigging snowing down here!!! I'm coming up to kill the frigging bastard who left the frigging milk in the frigging sun!!!" (You get the picture.)

The good news was...the pole crew had not crushed the sub against the rock. The bad news? The milk had curdled, and the water was so disgusting that words cannot describe it.

Fortunately, I was the person assigned to remove his hat and, probably because I was the oldest person on the set, I was protected from his wrath. "Jim," I explained, "just remember one thing. No one makes mistakes on purpose. You don't know the whole story."

We endured a long pause. Then, "Thanks Bob." And he retired to his trailer until Charlie had vacuumed up the curdled milk.

Our assistant director's helper was a cute and likeable young lady who had no idea fresh milk was cooling inside, that yesterday's milk had been destroyed by the sun, and that our assistant director would prefer suicide rather than pointing her out for blame. (As I said earlier, these were very pleasant people to work with and, fortunately, chivalry still survives!)

Our head electrician's name was Dwight, and everytime Cameron had a fit and began using his remarkable swear vocabulary, we would all turn our head in Dwight's direction for an evaluation. Our gaffer had measured Cameron's demeanor on a Richter Scale; a one meant next to nothing while a ten meant someone was going to be fired. The curdled milk episode measured at a nine, and when Mr. Cameron came to the surface, with the exception of his tender and his wife, every member of his troop was missing.

Scuba divers and remotely controlled miniatures were scattered everywhere, and it became quickly apparent that a method for filling the scuba bottles on the set was a necessity if we were to keep thirty divers in the water all day long. We ordered a large, electric, high-pressure compressor and, just to be sure, I ordered a dozen large bottles of breathing air and whips to plumb them together. Somehow, we kept up. Thank goodness Larry Smith was on the set as well.

At the end of the Coliseum shooting, Jim thanked us all. Just as he had observed everything else during the long shoot, he had not missed our taking over without being asked.

Following the film's debut, we had a party. As I waited to shake Cameron's hand, I overheard Andy, one of the electricians, tell Jim, "When I first met you, I thought you were a real asshole. However, you have won me over."

Most of the crew felt exactly the same way. But not me. I had liked and admired Jim Cameron from the very beginning, and I still do.

Twelve years have passed since the film, *The Abyss,* was released. Jim Cameron has made several films since then including *The Titanic.* During the making of this film, I waited for his little black Chevy convertible to turn onto my street; I imagined him begging me to help in the filming of that remarkable movie. But when he didn't show up, I realized we were simply business acquaintances, perhaps nothing else.

Then, serendipitously, Claudia and I attended the DEMA show, 2000, in Las Vegas. While ordering drinks before the dinner I looked up to see James Cameron standing beside us. He pumped my hand and gave Claudia a big hug. It meant a lot to both of us.

Mike was there as well, and we laughed remembering the filming of *The Abyss.* Jim confessed that the worst days of filming *The Titanic* were far easier than his best days on *The Abyss.*

A few months ago while I was working on this book, I heard rotor blades slapping high above. The roar was soon followed by a phone call. "Bob Kirby," a familiar voice came over the wire. "It's me, Mike Cameron. I'm at the airport. Let's have lunch and then you can fly Jim's helicopter."

During our flight I asked Mike how much the machine cost to operate. He didn't know, but he assumed it was a staggering amount.

My reply?

"Good."

FATE

I left my warm house, not knowing my fate
To enter the water, it was now getting late.
The pusher was mad, he was always that way,
Keeping me angered and forever at bay.
Dark, swirling liquid, lots of black mud,
Filled with things that make bone-chilling thuds.
I knew my task, to be under the pipe,
To jet it down till I'm dead and ripe.
Why am I here, and not in the sack,
With my warm, loving wife pressed tight to my back?
The answer is plain,
It is simply God's fate,
My time to enter
The Pearly Gate.

Fate or luck? What is the difference? I believe fate is unavoidable; God's wish, both good and bad. Luck, however, can be the same thing. This supplies me with a rather fuzzy answer. The story of my life.

Had I not had the luck of overhearing Jerry Todd and Nasty Ed discussing diving in the Ocean Beach restaurant in 1955, I would have ended up someplace else. Chances are I would not have become an abalone diver and devoted my life to the sea. I doubt I would have met Claudia, our two sons would not have been born, and neither would our loving grandchildren.

When I stop and think about it, the subject of fate and luck makes chills run up and down my back. I might never have experienced such an interesting life.

As I run my fingers over the keys of this one-eyed computer, my thoughts are somber, not humorous. So many of my old diving buddies have vanished into the big decompression tank in the sky and, since I am approaching seventy, my turn may be next. Consequently, it seems appropriate that I complete this book and, by setting my story straight, leave my grandchildren and those who follow them insight into my past and their generic fate — their future.

We massage our thoughts and, emulating our friends and relatives, our personalities are formed through encounters with others whom we admire, and some whom we don't particularly admire. We can't, however, change our God-given talents. (One of my grandsons, for example, shows clerical attributes while I possess absolutely no ability in this area.)

This book covers one area of my life with − believe it or not − some of the more brutal (adventuresome?) events eliminated. I have ignored my flamboyant years in the aviation industry. That story will have to wait for a second book.

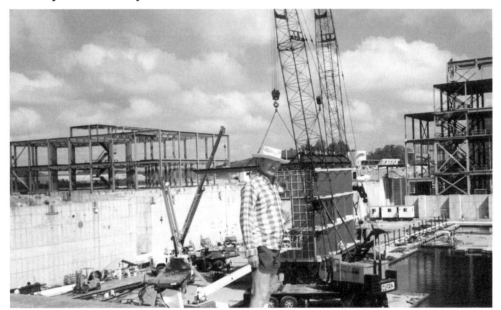

UGLY ME

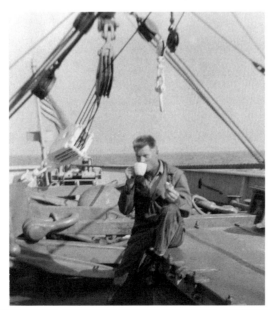

BOB DRINKING COFFEE ON NAVY SHIP, OCTOBER 1956

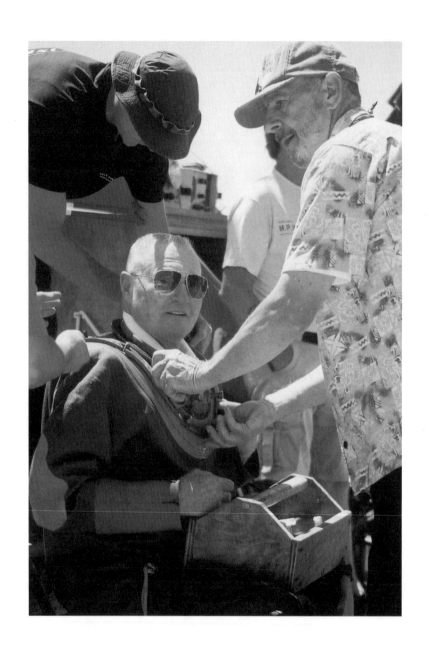

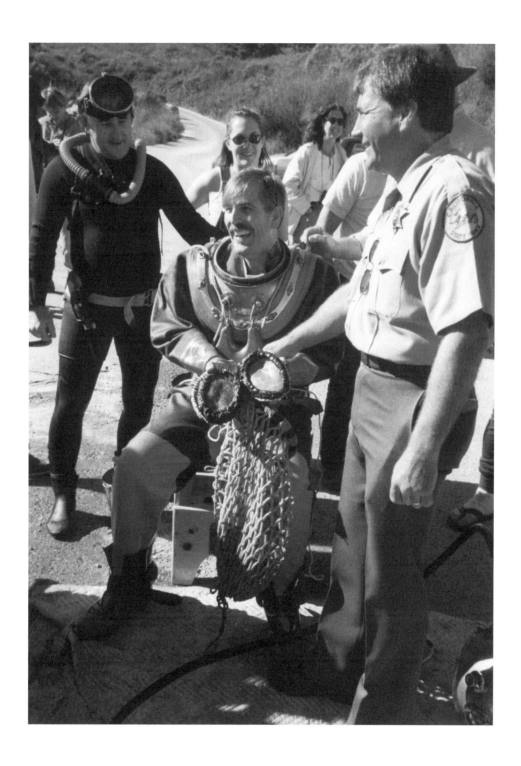

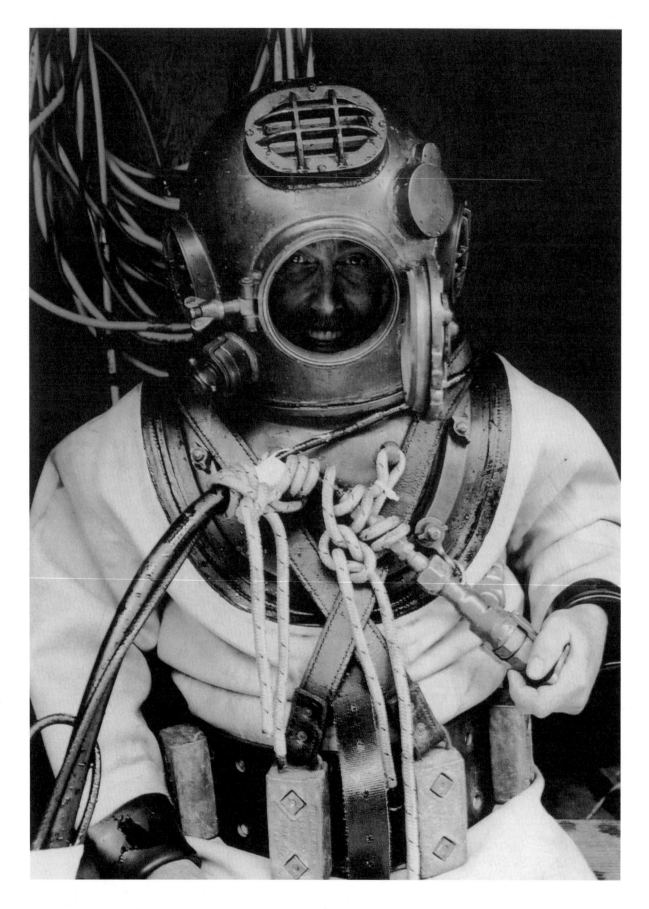

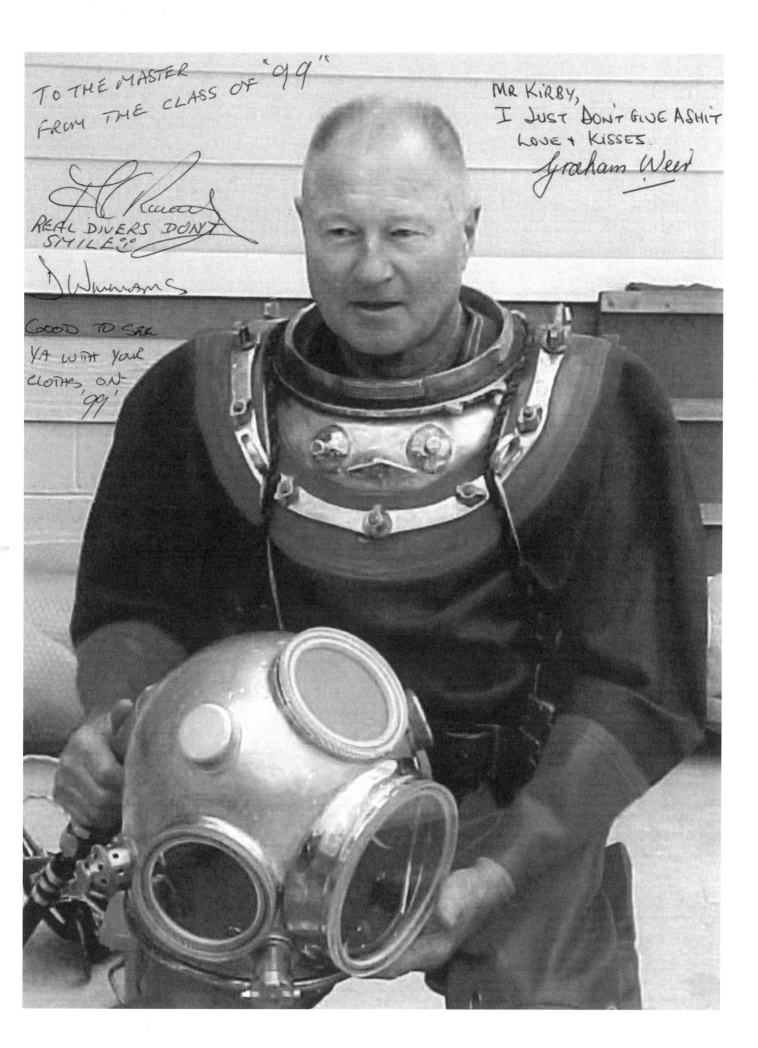

TO THE MASTER
FROM THE CLASS OF "99"

REAL DIVERS DON'T
SMILE!!

J Williams

GOOD TO SEE
YA WITH YOUR
CLOTHES ON
'99'

MR KIRBY,
I JUST DON'T GIVE A SHIT.
LOVE + KISSES.
Graham West

The Adventurer

You can keep your tame world of rockingchair life
I'll thrive in my world of challenge and strife
Once you've lived on the edge you can never go back
To sedentary ways of comfort and slack

I have no regrets though my path be uncertain
I open each window and draw back each curtain
And deal with the view whether pleasant or grim
My vision stays sharp though the picture be dim

The timid may think that I'm ruthless or coarse
But they choose to walk while I ride my own horse
To hell with the crowd, they all cling together
I've loosed all my bonds and cut free my tether

G.G. Ainsworth